Turning Evidence into Everyday Practice

An interim report from the PACE programme, November 1997

PACE team: Michael Dunning, Gerrard Abi-Aad,
David Gilbert, Steve Gillam, Hayley Livett

King's Fund

Published by
King's Fund Publishing
11–13 Cavendish Square
London W1M 0AN

© King's Fund 1998

First published 1998

ISBN 1 85717 151 9

A CIP catalogue record for this book is available from the British Library

Distributed by Grantham Book Services Ltd
Isaac Newton Way, Alma Park Industrial Estate, Grantham,
Lincolnshire NG31 9SD
Tel: 01476 541080
Fax: 01476 541061

Typeset by WordWise, Lee-on-the-Solent, Hampshire

Printed and bound in Great Britain by
The Looseleaf Company, Melksham, Wilts.

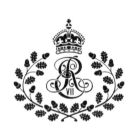

WX 20

WX 154.2
EVIDENCE BASED H/C ?
OUTCOM ASSES
EVAL STUDIES
COST EFFECT
QUALITY HEALTH CARE
NHS
CLINICAL AUDIT

Contents

Annexes

Introduction

The Promoting Action on Clinical Effectiveness (PACE) programme was set up in autumn 1995 and until now we have reported on the emerging lessons from the work as we have gone along. Circulation of regular *PACE Bulletins* – simple one-page notes about progress – and the preparation of a series of PACE discussion papers are part of this approach.

This interim report provides a more detailed review of progress. It describes the lessons from the work so far drawn from experiences from the local projects. We hope that these experiences will offer ideas to others engaged in implementing clinical effectiveness. It also identifies a series of current challenges being tackled in the projects. Examples of these are how to sustain service improvements secured initially through the local project work and how to ensure that clinical effectiveness becomes a normal way of practice within health service organisations.

The report is in six main parts:

Chapter 1 – provides some background notes about PACE
Chapter 2 – provides an overall report on progress in the projects
Chapter 3 – identifies the lessons from the projects so far
Chapter 4 – describes our approach to measuring the impact of the projects
Chapter 5 – describes some current challenges facing the projects.

And, finally:

Chapter 6 – reports on progress in the PACE Network.

In addition, there are several annexes which provide further details about the work so far.

This working report is based on a mid-term review undertaken in July 1997 – about half way through the programme – with colleagues involved in the local PACE projects. The work described here reflects their skill, enthusiasm and determination in taking these projects forward.

Michael Dunning, Gerrard Abi-Aad,
David Gilbert, Steve Gillam, Hayley Livett

Summary

This report is based on the work taken forward in the 16 projects between mid-1996 and mid-1997. *Change in practice is achievable* is the clear message from these experiences, but that encouraging view requires some qualification. Working to promote clinical effectiveness is complex and requires:

- Careful preparation, ensuring that those leading the work understand local factors that may influence progress

- Effective communications, ensuring that those likely to be affected by the work are kept in touch with progress

- Robust arrangements for managing the work and co-ordinating a range of contributions.

The experiences have also brought into sharper focus a number of challenges that will need resolution if work on clinical effectiveness is to have a lasting influence on health and health care:

- How to ensure that action to change clinical practice is matched by action to secure changes in service provision. It is pointless encouraging GPs to change their referral practice if secondary care cannot meet the increased demand for services

- How to ensure that improvements secured through the project work endure rather than fade away after the project has ended

- How to ensure that patients are able to play a full role in implementation

- How to ensure that clinical effectiveness becomes a normal way of working within health service organisations. This is likely to require integration of local systems and processes, such as audit, education and information services. Better integration will support implementation and ensure that the significant sums invested in these activities provide appropriate return.

Relationships between three groups may be essential for success in these endeavours:

- Clinicians – who need to be encouraged to see clinical effectiveness as part of continuing professional development

- Managers and policy makers – who need to play an active role in creating organisations within which clinical effectiveness can flourish

- Patients – who have a right to effective care.

Chapter 1

About PACE

Background

Since the early 1990s there has been growing interest in using the results of research to improve health and health services. This work has been taken forward under titles such as 'evidence-based practice', 'clinical effectiveness' and 'implementation of research findings'. Underlying these titles is a common concern to improve the quality of clinical decision making. Interest in this work has been stimulated by:

- Improved access to the results of research and improvements in the quality of reviews of primary research following the establishment of the UK Cochrane Centre (Oxford) and the Centre for Reviews and Dissemination (York)

- Variations in the level and quality of health care provision

- Concern to secure a return on the investment in research and development.

Initiatives have tended to focus either on professional development – helping individual clinicians to use research evidence as part of their clinical decision making – or organisational development designed to secure the implementation of evidence for a specific clinical condition. The work of the Centre for Evidence-Based Practice in Oxford is an example of the former; PACE is an example of the latter.

The PACE approach

There are three linked objectives for the PACE programme:

- To support 16 *local projects* within health authorities and NHS trusts in England to demonstrate the effective implementation of evidence-based practice

- To support a *network* of individuals who have an interest in clinical effectiveness

- To *disseminate* the lessons from the local projects.

The starting point for PACE was the Getting Research into Practice and Purchasing (GRiPP) project launched in Oxford in 1993. This project explored how health authorities could use research evidence in their commissioning role to improve health. GRiPP developed a series of steps, starting with the selection of topics for attention, that run through a local process of consultation and developing, disseminating and implementing evidence-based guidelines.

Similar work, the Framework for Appropriate Care Throughout Sheffield (FACTS) project, was launched in Sheffield in 1994. This project, focused on primary care, sought to create a quality controlled framework for changing clinical behaviour across one district.

These and other projects demonstrated the dearth of evidence about means of securing changes in clinical behaviour. A review of priorities for research on methods for securing the implementation of research findings was commissioned under the NHS R&D Programme (1996) and a programme of research is now in hand. The Cochrane Collaboration on Effective Professional Practice (CCEPP) also leads an extensive programme of systematic reviews of primary research on changing clinical behaviour. A series of reviews will be published by CCEPP in 1998. A guide to some key references and resources related to methods of implementation is in Annex 1c.

In developing the PACE programme the emphasis has been on 'action learning'. Those leading the local projects have adapted different techniques for change to local circumstances, and adopted a process of reflection within their own teams. The available evidence suggests that intensive efforts using a set of linked interventions are more likely to be successful, so the focus has been on developing an integrated approach to implementing change. The programme is supported by the NHS Executive; local projects received a grant (£30,000 over two years) to support the work and cover some of the incidental costs.

The PACE programme has been taken forward within a framework that:

- Ensures that the individual projects are not isolated and creates a process to enable them to work together through regular meetings of representatives from all the 16 local projects

- Allows people involved in similar endeavours to learn from the work as the projects develop and the lessons from the work emerge through membership of the PACE Network

- Enables anyone who is interested to keep in touch with the work through the *PACE Bulletin*.

Evaluation

Evaluation of the PACE programme involves:

- *Identifying lessons learnt*. There is a regular dialogue between the PACE team and local projects. In addition a series of PACE Project Group meetings, involving representatives of all the 16 projects, ensure that lessons are identified and captured in ways that facilitate their dissemination

- Support to the projects to help them *measure the impact* of what they have changed. Measurement is a complex element of all the local projects. Reflecting the diversity of the clinical topics being addressed, reliance on a single data source would not be plausible or practical. The projects will influence a number of clinical activities such as diagnostic testing, prescribing patterns and treatments. The aim has been therefore to identify a basket of measures that, when taken together, can reliably indicate the trend and scale of change. A set of principles to guide this work has been identified (*see* Chapter 4)

● An *external evaluation* is being undertaken by a team based at Templeton College, Oxford. This provides an independent means of assessing how the changes have been achieved by the local projects and the influence of the King's Fund management of the programme overall. The results of the early stages of this work are reflected in this report and further findings will feed into future publications about PACE.

Contact details for the PACE team are in Annex 1a.

Annex 1b provides lists of issues of *PACE Bulletin* and PACE discussion papers.

Chapter 2

Progress on the Projects

Arrangements for the selection of the 16 projects were completed in April 1996 and pen-pictures of the projects are in Annex 2a. Projects were selected against three broad criteria:

- The project needed to be of *high priority* locally, with support from senior levels within key local organisations

- The work had to be based on *robust evidence*

- There needed to be sound proposals for *managing the work*.

Sixteen sites were chosen that reflect a broad range of clinical topics, types of intervention and settings. By June 1997, twelve months into the work, the projects reported progress in several areas. This chapter provides a broad description of progress so far.

Preparing the ground

Each project has a project leader within a local team to take the work forward. In some cases an existing staff member acted as project co-ordinator, while in others an external appointment was made for this role. A local senior steering or advisory group was also created to oversee the project work. In many cases the project built on existing work, either on clinical effectiveness or on a related clinical topic.

The team was always multi-disciplinary, seeking to incorporate and represent the main stakeholders involved – clinicians, therapists, managers and, when possible, patients or their representatives (such as Community Health Council members). If patients were not directly involved in the project team, most projects sought to explore how they could be involved. The role of different clinicians and health professionals, for example pharmacists and physiotherapists, was vital. Non-clinical staff, from information technology services to portering, were also involved.

In some cases, multi-disciplinary work went one step further to multi-agency work involving, for example, social services. Even without the explicit engagement of such agencies, the work has implications for health and social care, acute services and the community, and can cross the boundaries between curative and preventive activities.

The next step was agreeing on a project plan to ensure a coherent view of how the change process was to be managed. To help this process, the project team had to gain an understanding of where they were starting from. This involved understanding current clinical practice, identifying information sources and communication channels (or developing them) and setting up monitoring processes that would provide baseline data. It also meant identifying key local opinion leaders whose involvement was likely to be important to the smooth delivery of the project plan.

Much effort was spent on securing local consensus over the relevance and interpretation of research evidence, including the formulation of local guidelines or care pathways. In many cases, professionals from different research traditions and with varying attitudes towards the nature of evidence had to be accommodated.

Securing action

The projects planned a variety of activities and interventions to ensure that the research evidence and proposals for change were communicated as effectively as possible. Several projects set about early development of local education programmes to support the dissemination of local guidelines. Various ways of engaging clinicians have been tried, including the use of incentives (such as accreditation to attend meetings) to encourage clinical change.

The work implied a balance of activities across primary and secondary care and the use of mechanisms for achieving change, such as:

- Development of guidelines, protocols and care pathways

- Educational programmes

- Employment of a project facilitator

- Information packs for clinicians

- Targeted mailings to doctors

- Newsletters

- Patient focus groups

- Patient information materials

- Media campaigns

- Co-option of other professionals (such as pharmacists) to encourage change

- Development of networks around common interests.

The main emphasis has been on educational and developmental work with correspondingly less emphasis on more costly interventions – such as one-to-one academic detailing or financial incentives. At the same time, the projects had to cope with personnel changes, professional tensions and the need for effective project management.

Making time for the project as a whole is a continuing challenge. Material produced as part of the local work, and which is available from the project leaders, is listed in Annex 2a.

Barriers and obstacles

There were many barriers and obstacles to overcome as the projects were taken forward – it was not all plain sailing. Much of the early effort was in planning and preparation. In some projects, attempting to balance and prioritise various aspects of the workload proved difficult. An environment of continual change within some organisations, (whether of staff or senior management or due to restructuring), meant a lack of continuity in the project work. These situations made planning for service consequences even more difficult. Where projects were developed within a wider programme, this could overcome some of the sense of isolation and help anchor it within the organisation. Projects sometimes had difficulties identifying stakeholders and their interests.

Some of the barriers to change, identified in discussion during 1996, are listed below. They are described in more detail in Annex 2b. This list is taken from the PACE discussion paper *Getting Started* (September 1996):

● Lack of perception of relevance

● Lack of resources

● Short-term outlook

● Conflicting priorities

● The difficulty in measuring outcomes

● Lack of necessary skills

● No history of multi-disciplinary working

● Limitations of the research evidence on effectiveness

● Perverse incentives

● Intensity of contribution required.

Chapter 3

PACE: The Lessons so far

This chapter describes the lessons so far and draws on examples from work in the 16 projects.

A. Preparing the ground

Careful preparation to promote a common understanding of the aim is an essential precursor to the launch of local initiatives. This could include work on the specific topic (for example, in assembling a picture of current practice and drawing together the evidence) or organisation-wide discussions to promote clinical effectiveness. Criteria to guide the selection of topics for attention locally could include:

- The strength of evidence

- The magnitude of change required

- The scale of support for the changes required

- Potential benefit for patients.

Many obstacles are likely to be encountered when promoting work on clinical effectiveness, so clarity about the purpose of the work and the likely benefits will be important. The initiative might be regarded in a variety of ways, for example: as part of a cost-cutting exercise; as a managerial intervention intended to reduce clinical freedom; or as part of a single-minded drive to implement a single piece of evidence

Lesson A1
Base local guidelines on national reviews of evidence and guidelines

It is more efficient to take forward work on a base of evidence offered by material (such as guidelines or systematic reviews) produced by reputable national and regional bodies, rather than to seek to replicate the review process locally. A comprehensive search for reputable guidelines should therefore be undertaken as a first step.

Building on such material can clarify which elements of subsequent local guidelines are evidence-based and which are consensus-based. The process is likely to be welcomed by many clinicians. These local discussions can help to secure ownership of the guidelines.

Examples:

The Bradford *H. pylori* eradication project found that GPs preferred evidence-based guidelines to those based on clinical opinion.

The timetable for the Dorset menorrhagia project meant that the team was developing its own guidelines in parallel to a review being undertaken by the Royal College of

Obstetricians and Gynaecologists. Availability of the latter could have speeded up the local discussions.

The Southern Derbyshire back pain project has been able to build local discussions on the Clinical Standards Advisory Group (CSAG) report on back pain.

Lesson A2
Acknowledge that evidence may be ambiguous and incomplete

People unfamiliar with research evidence may have unrealistic expectations about what it offers. Even thorough systematic reviews may need careful translation to enable research to be applied in an everyday practice setting. It is important therefore to acknowledge uncertainties about evidence. There are many questions the evidence may not answer – for example, about the most cost-effective model of service delivery.

Examples:

The Barnet hypertension project found that, while general evidence is available related to hypertension, there are major gaps concerning thresholds for treatment and risk management approaches for ethnic groups.

The Dorset menorrhagia project noted that very few procedures are 100% effective and clinicians need to explain uncertainty to patients.

Lesson A3
Be clear about what needs to change

Do not launch into the creation of local guidelines as a first step. Clarity about the nature of current practice provides an essential backdrop to discussions about the need for change and, for example, the need to formulate a local guideline. Questions to address include:

- Have all existing relevant local guidelines been identified?

- What problems were encountered in seeking their implementation?

- Have all recent relevant audits been reviewed?

- What are the main perceived deficiencies in service delivery?

Examples:

In the Bromley *H. pylori* eradication project, discussions on developing guidelines made little progress until clinical scenarios to illustrate current practice were produced. These allowed the local group to bring current practice and evidence side by side and focused questions on divergent practice. This generated debate and enthusiasm for change.

The Wigan and Bolton continence project used audits to highlight problems with the current standards of care and demonstrate the merit in developing guidelines.

Lesson A4
Link the work into local priorities

Health care organisations are constantly evolving in response to a wide range of social, demographic and political influences. Many factors are therefore likely to influence the choice of local priorities. Similarly, many issues influence what is important to primary health care teams.

It is important to keep under review how the work is presented locally and how coherence with local priorities is maintained. This means that questions about service and resource consequences can be addressed in health authority commissioning plans and trust development plans. Before new initiatives are launched, find out whether the topic was an issue in previous plans and understand the results of any initiative.

Examples:

The Lambeth, Southwark and Lewisham and King's Health Care cardiac rehabilitation project was able to build on links with a wider programme of work on Implementing Clinical Effectiveness (ICE), which had the support of the health authority and local NHS trusts.

The Royal Berkshire leg ulcer project was launched when the main concern was about quality of clinical care. Later, concern about the costs of surgical supplies provided an opportunity to emphasise the likely cost savings from the project and reinforce organisational commitment to the project.

Lesson A5
Consider the options available for securing change

There has been much attention nationally and locally to questions about methods of securing change in clinical behaviour, for example, through the work of CCEPP (*see* Chapter 1 and Annex 1c). A list of the mechanisms being used by the local projects is in Chapter 2.

Issues involved in changing clinical practice are increasingly the subject of research. It would be wise to be up to date on this knowledge and review the options available before initiating development projects. The expertise established through similar projects elsewhere can also provide sources of advice.

Lesson A6
Understand local issues and potential barriers to change

Consider carefully who is likely to be affected by the work and ensure that their concerns are understood. Clarity about likely objections and resistance to change will facilitate project planning. The work may be seen as threatening by some clinicians and action may need to be taken to overcome these fears. Essential early steps are to identify the key local individuals and secure their support (these could include consultants and other specialists, clinical directors, influential GPs, postgraduate tutors, nurse educators, nurse managers, influential managers and clinical audit managers). It is important to identify also those individuals whose support – as leaders of local opinion – may be critical to success.

Examples:

The Dudley continence project found that staff from their successful pilot sites could act as 'product champions' – taking the message to others.

The Royal Berkshire leg ulcer project saw the need to identify and negotiate with 'gatekeepers' – clinicians with sufficient influence and authority to affect the outcome of decision making, although not necessarily taking part in direct clinical care.

The Wirral family support in schizophrenia project linked a family support worker with a community psychiatric team. Later discussions indicated that earlier involvement of other local interests, such as social services, would have been beneficial (*see* Annex 3c).

Lesson A7
Take into account the needs and interests of GPs and primary health care teams

Pharmaceutical companies have developed ways of analysing practice-specific information to help with marketing programmes. This approach recognises that practices will have their own interests and pressures and it is unrealistic to expect all practices to embrace new information at the same pace.

Experience from the PACE projects has confirmed the need to build on the diversity of primary care. Sources of information about primary care could include locality commissioning teams, medical and pharmaceutical advisers, GP tutors and educational networks. Plans for local implementation projects should build on this intelligence and develop a programme to engage practices gradually – starting with those likely to adopt new approaches.

Examples:

The Bromley *H. pylori* eradication project commented that 'you need as many plans as practices'.

The North Derbyshire congestive cardiac failure project found that working with practice managers through their regular meetings was an effective, non-clinical way to initiate work with practices.

The Southern Derbyshire back pain project is exploring how information locally available, about general practices, can help expand their education programme.

Annex 3b is adapted from a special issue of the *PACE Bulletin* (June 1997) about working with primary care.

Lesson A8
Establish data required to monitor progress

Inaccuracies in routine information systems are likely to hamper the evaluation of local clinical effectiveness initiatives. Moreover, the lack of information technology systems that integrate clinical audit into day-to-day practice is a major hurdle. These problems can be overcome if ways are found to harness information from a range of systems. A basket of measures taken together can enable measurement of progress. Sources of data include prescription analysis and cost (PACT) data, contract minimum data sets (MDS), existing performance indicator (PI) packages, any local disease registers and the local hospital patient administration systems (PAS).

Example:

The Walsall *H. pylori* eradication project recorded that one of the most important lessons was the need to establish – at the start of the project – an agreement with all those involved for systems and procedures to collect and analyse data.

See also the examples in Chapter 4.

B. Securing action

Experience is showing that carefully constructed programmes, which build on what is known about securing changes in clinical behaviour, can be successful. The project plans cover work over two years (from summer 1996) but already some changes to clinical practice and services have been achieved. Many of the projects have pilot phases to help them understand what works locally.

Lesson B1
Present the change in terms of benefits for staff and patients

Be clear about what will change for staff and patients. Promote the idea that the objective is to incorporate changes into routine clinical practice rather than create new and additional work. However, do acknowledge that in the short term some additional effort might be required. Incentives could include a fast-track referral to the consultant and the award of educational recognition for the work.

Examples:

The Bradford, Bromley and Walsall *H. pylori* eradication projects should, in the longer term, reduce repeat prescriptions and eradicate peptic ulcer disease in a significant number of patients.

The Wirral family support in schizophrenia project should take some pressure off GPs.

Lesson B2
Help people work together

All the projects involve some degree of multi-disciplinary working. The development of evidence-based practice can provide a valuable catalyst to the creation of effectively performing teams. A strong team culture can provide a climate within which more cautious members can be encouraged to move along with the others. Clarity about roles and contributions need to be established. Careful thought needs to be given to the membership of teams, which may need to involve clinicians and managers. A good understanding of team dynamics and good facilitation skills can help the development of local teams.

Examples:

The Bradford *H. pylori* eradication project found that local discussions about the project strengthened relationships and partnerships between clinicians, particularly between consultants and GPs.

The establishment of the Gloucester management of stroke patients project (which built on the work of an existing group of therapists) meant new members being brought into the group from other disciplines. The rapid expansion of people involved took time to work through. This also exposed differences in research tradition between the different disciplines, which were overcome by promoting debates about various research methodologies.

Lesson B3
Provide a local education and training programme

Educational programmes are an essential element of all local projects. There is extensive literature about professional learning and personal development and how to create suitable programmes (*see* Annex 1c). Questions to address include:

● Does the programme reflect the needs of individuals and organisations?

● Should the programme be multi-disciplinary?

● Can staff be released to attend?

● Does the programme attract professional recognition?

Examples:

The Oxfordshire post-operative pain control project is having to overcome problems encountered in arranging group training for nurses, because there was no mechanism for providing clinical cover.

An approach for assessing training needs has been developed as part of the South Tyne stable angina project, to support an educational programme for practice and community nurses. A personal development plan allows participants to monitor their own learning and facilitate the later audit of the educational programme. The model is being extended to cover medical staff.

The Wigan and Bolton continence project found that their training sessions provided a valuable means of building relationships between staff in different local trusts and primary health care teams. Training is being provided for community pharmacists so that they can offer advice to patients consistent with the advice given by NHS staff.

Lesson B4
Give more than information to primary health care teams

Providing information alone to primary health care teams is unlikely to secure significant change in practice. Some GPs may adopt new guidelines but the majority may carry on as before. With many projects one of the key steps has been to change the nature of care and treatment for existing patients. Many projects provided someone to select patients from practice records whose condition falls within the scope of the new guidelines and establishing arrangements with the GP to review their treatment.

Deploying a project co-ordinator, to work with practice nurses, has proved to be helpful in several projects. This approach helps to build in continuity so that the records can be maintained in ways that facilitate regular monitoring. Other important supports are educational material, educational approval of the programme, identification of support networks and advice about information technology systems.

Examples:

In the Bromley *H. pylori* eradication project, the local project team worked with practices to identify existing patients whose treatment appeared to merit review in the light of the new guidelines.

The Lambeth, Southwark and Lewisham and King's Health Care cardiac rehabilitation project found that records of repeat prescriptions were a practical way of identifying existing patients.

Lesson B5
A balanced approach across primary and secondary care is important

Many of the local projects will affect the interaction between primary and secondary care and have required an even-handed approach to ensure progress – for example, by not trying to change primary care in isolation.

Example:

The introduction by the Walsall *H. pylori* eradication project of a local guideline, focused on clinical management in primary care, led to a review of hospital referrals.

Lesson B6
Decide how to engage pharmaceutical companies

Changes to prescribing practice are aims for many PACE projects and a local policy about handling links with pharmaceutical companies is important. There are dangers that local representatives may offer conflicting advice and information in their contacts with local clinicians. Questions may also arise about the supply of staff or equipment by companies. Before embarking on dialogue with local companies be clear about whether you need to engage them and what the benefits and risks are. Resolution of some of these issues will require negotiating skills and an understanding about the working methods of pharmaceutical companies.

Example:

In the North Derbyshire congestive cardiac failure project a written agreement about the nature and scope of the work was established at senior level (between the local company director and the health authority chief executive). The agreement was to support activities but not to promote their products and secured the use of a mobile echo machine and support for educational activities. A potential problem of a company using the project to promote its product was resolved in part because of the existence of such an agreement.

C. Managing the work

Work to promote clinical effectiveness is complex and time-consuming. It needs the development of partnerships and communications across different organisational boundaries and within them. It also means keeping those affected by the work informed about what is going on.

Lesson C1
Create a realistic timetable

It is easy to be too ambitious in drawing up a project plan and overlook the time required for essential parts of the task. The individual elements of the work require detailed attention – for example, to appraise evidence and to consult across a range of health service organisations. It is also difficult for clinical staff to balance this work with their clinical responsibilities.

Questions to address include:

- Has the timetable been synchronised with other relevant activities, such as the development of commissioning plans?

- Have all the main players agreed the significant dates?

- Has the timetable been explained to those likely to be affected by the work?

Examples:

The Gloucester Royal Infirmary management of stroke patients project encountered problems in maintaining a timetable when clinical staff were coping with staff shortages and seasonal variations in medical emergencies.

The South Tyne stable angina project emphasised that the project group was likely to undertake most of the work. Balancing this work with clinical responsibilities was difficult. Dedicated time was required.

The Walsall *H. pylori* eradication project underestimated the time necessary to design and produce materials such as referral pro formas and guidelines.

The Wigan and Bolton continence project underestimated the problem of getting the project discussed at key local meetings where the agendas are fixed months in advance.

Lesson C2
Decide how to co-ordinate the work

All the projects are led from senior level within organisations (nursing director, general practitioner, consultant physician, director of public health, consultant in public health medicine). In addition, most projects also chose to appoint someone as a project co-ordinator to handle the day-to-day work. There were some attractions for redeploying an existing member of staff for this role, for example familiarity with local systems and services. This can create some problems, such as when the co-ordinator continues to be identified with his/her previous post. Another project has shown that someone with the necessary skills and experience but appointed from elsewhere can be effective. One project learnt how difficult it was, without a co-ordinator, to maintain momentum on the project while trying to fit the work in with other business.

It has usually proved invaluable to have someone with dedicated responsibility for the day-to-day project tasks. It would be sensible to identify and review the advantages and disadvantages of the main options available before making final plans.

Lesson C3
Recognise that new skills may be required

Experience has reaffirmed the range of skills needed to manage work on clinical effectiveness, such as the use of critical appraisal skills, techniques for managing change, managing clinical audit and the development and delivery of local educational programmes. Some of these skills may be new to those involved. Before launching new initiatives it would be helpful to identify locally available skills, establish how they can contribute to the work, and decide how to remedy any important deficiencies.

Examples:

Clinicians in two NHS trusts have taken responsibility for the Oxfordshire post-operative pain control project. They have found the experience challenging and rewarding, as they have developed project management skills.

Having a team member in the Royal Berkshire leg ulcer project with facilitation skills has enabled meetings and the work more generally to proceed smoothly.

Lesson C4
Keep in touch with those affected by the work

Effective communications have been essential:

- Within the project team

- With the local senior steering group

- With other local interests affected by the work, including clinicians and patients.

It seems best to use existing local networks and communications routes rather than creating new and untested approaches. Providing written information is not a substitute for the spoken word. Face-to-face meetings are a better way to promote true involvement. Any written information provided to team members, clinicians and patients needs to be standardised and clear, and should provide contact details and sources of further information.

Examples:

The Dudley continence project found that personal contact was more successful than formal meetings. They also linked local publicity to a National Continence Day.

The Oxfordshire post-operative pain control project found that there were no channels to communicate clinical protocols to a rapidly changing workforce so specific arrangements had to be made for the project.

In the Royal Berkshire leg ulcer project a strategy was agreed to help overcome the difficulties in managing communications: there were doubts about creating yet another local newsletter! This strategy places responsibility on individual members of the project advisory group to ensure that they maintain contact and relay information to individual groups (for example, practice nurses).

Annex 3c is adapted from a PACE discussion paper (March 1997) about effective communications.

Lesson C5
Retain a balanced approach

The projects planned to incorporate a range of activities, including assessment of evidence, development of guidelines, educational programmes and work with patients. A balanced approach avoids over-concentration on specific elements. For example, avoid devoting too much time to the development and presentation of a local guideline – this may be the easy part of the task. Other tasks, in particular education and training, could have more impact in securing change.

Example:

The Lambeth, Southwark and Lewisham and King's Health Care cardiac rehabilitation project realised at one stage that its work with patients had become separated from other elements of the work and prevented them influencing one another. It has since taken steps to ensure a more coherent approach.

Lesson C6
Do not be too ambitious

The evidence base may represent a small part of the knowledge required to develop comprehensive guidelines for specific health conditions. Evidence will therefore have to be complemented with consensus opinion about good practice. It may be best to start in the area where there is robust evidence and plan an incremental programme to adopt consensus guidelines once the first (evidence-based) element has been changed. A focus on what is achievable within a realistic timetable is sensible.

Example:

The initial plan in the South Tyne stable angina project to develop guidelines and implement a comprehensive approach to angina management has proved to be over-ambitious. It was decided to delay work on some aspects, such as lifestyle advice on exercise levels and patient satisfaction surveys.

Lesson C7
Expect the unexpected and be able to respond

However carefully project plans are compiled, recognise a need for flexibility. A range of events may conspire to delay the work. For example, it is unwise to rely heavily on one person; develop a team approach so that team members share the work.

Examples:

A number of personnel changes over the first half of the Chase Farm pressure sore management project has reinforced the need to avoid over-reliance on one person.

The Dudley continence project found it was important to adapt the project to the different ways that local primary health care teams worked and not be overly prescriptive about the way things should be done.

The original plan in the Lambeth, Southwark and Lewisham and King's Health Care cardiac rehabilitation project envisaged an outreach nurse working with patients in the community but this was changed to include development work with practices. This led to more rapid progress.

The lessons described above are listed in Annex 3a.

Chapter 4

Evaluation: Measuring Impact

Guiding principles

From the start, the PACE team and local projects agreed principles to guide work on measuring impact:

- Rely on *original research* and do not try to replicate primary research

- Focus on *the process of implementation* rather than on health outcomes

- Rely wherever possible on *routine data sources*

- Identify *suitable comparisons*

- Establish a *baseline* against which to measure impact

- Build in a process to *monitor progress*

- Keep it *as simple as possible.*

Subsequent discussions established a group of indicators for each local project. Progress is being made in the assembly of baseline data and in ensuring a monitoring process. The principles listed above are described in more detail in Annex 4a.

Examples

The approach being adopted can be illustrated by the use of examples drawn from four projects (pen-pictures of the individual projects are in Annex 2a, including references to the evidence on which they are based). The information presented in this chapter is based on the actual data provided by various PACE projects. It is intended to illustrate an approach to measurement.

It is impossible at this stage to attribute any apparent change to the activities of the PACE programme. As more data become available, particularly comparative data, the issue of attribution will become clearer. The overall approach being adopted will be reflected in project reports due for completion in 1998.

1. North Derbyshire Health Authority – Congestive cardiac failure

Key measures:

- Prescribing ratio of loop diuretics to ACE inhibitors

- Admissions for heart failure

● Re-admissions for heart failure

● Reduction in mortality and morbidity.

This project is seeking to embed the effective management of heart failure by working closely with local primary and secondary care providers. Evidence suggests that a reduction of mortality and morbidity can be achieved through raising awareness and education on appropriate investigation and treatment of heart failure. An important element of this is to ensure appropriate prescribing of ACE inhibitors.

Figure 1 shows a favourable decline in the prescribing ratio between loop diuretics and anti-hypertensives, which include ACE inhibitors. Comparative information will be used to assess the significance of this change.

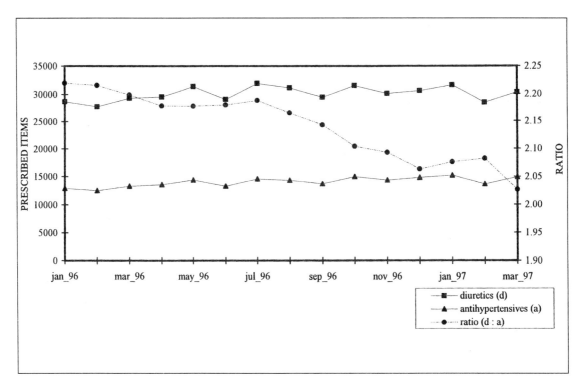

Figure 1 *North Derbyshire Health Authority: ratio of diuretic to anti-hypertensive prescribing (source: PACT). Note that ACE inhibitors are also used in the treatment of hypertension; changes in prescribing specifically for cardiac failure may be concealed by changes in prescribing in the management of hypertension.*

2. Bradford Health Authority – *Helicobacter pylori* eradication

Key measures:

● Trend in prescribing for ulcer-healing drugs

● Dose-specific trends in prescribing for clarithromycin and metronidazole

● Endoscopy rates

Bradford Health Authority is developing a co-ordinated approach to the effective management of patients with dyspepsia to ensure that:

- All existing patients known to have duodenal ulcer (DU) and who are on repeat H_2 antagonists are offered eradication therapy

- No patient with endoscopically proven DU is put on long-term H_2 antagonist treatment without being considered for *H. pylori* eradication.

Figure 2 below shows the trend in eradication therapy prescribing in twelve pilot practices before and after guideline dissemination and education. The rate of increase in the trend of prescribing, particularly of clarithromycin, provides an indication of a shift in GP behaviour in line with the evidence on eradication therapy. After a sufficient period of time a related decline in the trend of ulcer-healing drug prescribing (Figure 3, overleaf) should be detectable.

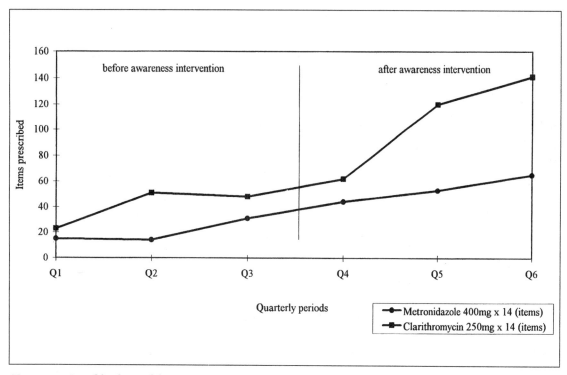

Figure 2 *Bradford Health Authority: dose-specific prescribing in pilot practices, a marker for triple therapy prescribing (source: PACT).*

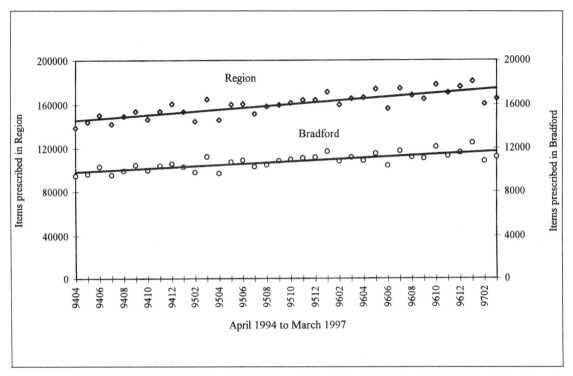

Figure 3 *Bradford Health Authority compared with Northern and Yorkshire Region: trend in ulcer-healing drug prescribing (source: PACT).*

3. Chase Farm Hospitals NHS Trust – Pressure sore management

Key measures:

● Decline in the proportion of ward-acquired pressure sores

● Trend in use of dressings

● Average length of stay

Prevention of pressure sores involves four key aspects:

● Improved education for all health professions

● The systematic identification of patients at risk of developing a sore, using a risk calculator

● A co-ordinated preventive plan of care with contribution from all health care professionals

● The selection of equipment needed to protect the patient whilst lying or sitting

In Figure 4 opposite the number of ward-acquired pressure sores is compared with the total number of reported pressure sores. The line (percentage ward-acquired) shows the percentage of pressure sores that are ward-acquired. Decline in the proportion of ward-acquired pressure sores closely accompanies the activities of the project team outlined above.

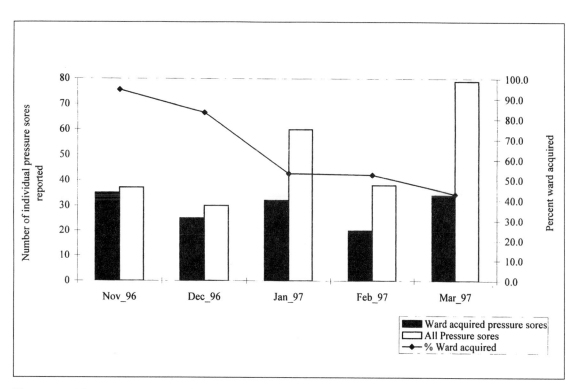

Figure 4 *Chase Farm Hospitals NHS Trust: pressure sore monitoring.*

4. South Tyneside Health Care Trust – The management of stable angina

Key measures:

- Aspirin and beta blocker prescribing patterns

- Hospital admissions for acute myocardial infarction (MI)

- Audit of the management of stable angina in primary care

South Tyneside has one of the highest mortality rates for ischaemic heart disease (IHD) in England and Wales. Over 30% of acute hospital admissions to South Tyneside District Hospital are IHD related. There is also local evidence that the management of patients with IHD is sub-optimal and not evidence-based.

The major objectives of the South Tyneside project are:

- To implement evidence-based guidelines for the management of chronic stable angina in primary and secondary care

- To improve the medical care of patients with IHD and to measure these changes.

Figure 5 overleaf shows the trend in the number of admissions for acute MI. This trend is being monitored against the trend in a neighbouring population to establish the effect of the programme on more serious forms of heart disease. Given the natural history of the disease process in this particular instance, it is not expected that any detectable change will occur over the timetable for the project.

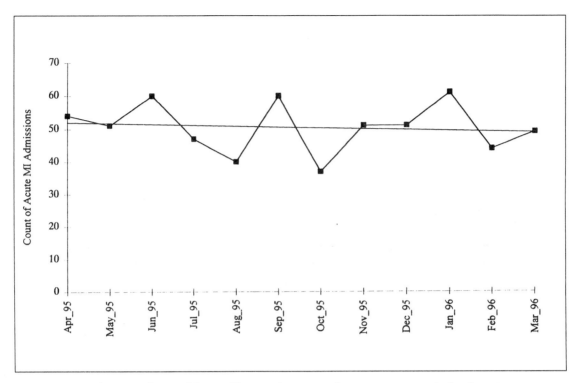

Figure 5 *South Tyneside Healthcare Trust: admissions for acute myocardial infarction.*

Measurement: some conclusions

Local projects have established mechanisms to collect and monitor indicators and the preliminary results are encouraging. However, it is too early to attribute any significance to the trends and a number of cautionary notes:

● Has change occurred because of the projects? The tension between the purism of a controlled experiment and the pragmatism required to ensure a co-ordinated approach to service development needs to be recognised. The group of indicators that has been identified for each project will complement the internal audits being carried out by many of the local projects and the independent evaluation by Templeton College

● The natural history of certain disease processes will complicate the detection of change. For example, in the management of stable angina it may be difficult to measure changes in mortality rates, given the short time frame and the progression of angina to more serious cardiac conditions

● The task of monitoring and data collection takes time and further discussions are required to establish how this task is best managed

● Routine data collection systems do not easily lend themselves to measuring impact of this kind. Solutions to overcome the limitations of routine data have been found. For example, in the case of *H. pylori* eradication, Bradford Health Authority is using dose specific monitoring of clarithromycin and metronidazole as a proxy indicator for triple therapy prescribing.

The assessment of the indicators for each project will help to establish a practical and reliable framework for measuring the impact of implementation activities. More work is required to build in appropriate comparisons and to examine the difference between project and comparison. How best to analyse the cost implications for the projects is another task under review.

Chapter 5

Current Challenges

The main challenges being addressed as the local projects are taken forward include the service and resources consequences of implementing change in clinical practice, sustaining change secured through the project work, involving patients in the work and generalising the lessons from the project work to ensure that the learning can be applied to other clinical topics.

Service and resource consequences

Ensuring that initiatives to change clinical practice are matched by action to secure funding for, and changes to services is proving to be one of the main challenges for many of the local projects.

Health economists argue that more effective practice is by definition cost saving. However, as one local project leader said: 'evidence-based practice costs money'. The cost pressures arise because changes to implement effective clinical practice may reduce health care costs within one defined area but may well raise them in another. Managing such cost transfers is a complex task.

Examples of the cost implications are:

- Increased referral activity – in North Derbyshire for echocardiography to manage congestive cardiac failure, in South Tyneside for exercise ECGs to manage angina and in Bromley for an increased number of endoscopies

- Increased prescribing costs – in Barnet for anti-hypertensives to prevent stroke and in Bradford, Bromley and Walsall for triple therapy to eradicate *H. pylori*. A rise in prescribing costs may cause problems for practices only towards the year end as PACT data reveal new financial pressures and the following year's prescribing budgets are set

- Increasing pressure to invest in new services – in Southern Derbyshire a rehabilitation service for sufferers of back pain to relieve pressure on physiotherapy waiting lists

- Increased work for audit staff – in many projects supporting retrospective audits in primary care.

An example of where costs are incurred in one sector in anticipation of later savings elsewhere is the case of more appropriate prescribing of ACE inhibitors (costlier now for GPs). In the longer term this should reduce hospitalisation rates among people with congestive cardiac failure (and reduce hospital costs).

Better ways of predicting service consequences may help. For example, modelling of the economic consequences of *H. pylori* eradication or better management of congestive cardiac failure should now be possible. This will help strengthen planning and the case for change. It will also provide data to monitor the impact of the local projects. Some costs that are difficult to predict are frequently overlooked – for example, the need to update guidelines or undertake re-audits.

Experience with the local projects has highlighted the importance of thinking through the likely service and resource consequences of new projects at the outset. Health authorities need to plan ahead rather than be presented with unplanned and unexpected increases in referrals, diagnostic or therapeutic activity. A link to the business planning, performance review and contracting cycles is therefore important. Staff in health authorities and NHS trusts who can secure the necessary financial commitment need to be involved in the discussions from an early stage.

Sustaining change

Many people involved in local projects have highlighted the difficulties of ensuring that changes to clinical practice as a consequence of the projects endure, so that today's innovation becomes tomorrow's routine practice.

A project approach to the management of tasks allows clarity about targets and timetables and a distinctiveness about the work that enables progress monitoring. Conversely, the dangers of a project approach are well known. A focused team with dedicated resources may have difficulty transferring their dedication and expertise to others. Projects are often launched with great enthusiasm; they secure change in the short term but the improvements may fade away after the project comes to an end.

Local project teams have learned – or relearned – basic principles of change management. Projects have flourished where a committed, influential team has managed to communicate a vision of what it is trying to achieve. Most of the likely forces for and against change can be anticipated. Many project teams have sought to weave their work into the resources already available locally to secure change, for example, clinical audit and professional development. The progress of some projects has been eased where audit and effectiveness are not seen as separate initiatives. This is clearly easier where the same management teams are involved. This close alignment with local systems may help ensure that the changes endure.

Some of the issues that may need to be resolved are:

● Promoting a *wider view of clinical effectiveness*: the work tends to be regarded as 'clinical business' and a matter to be taken forward solely by doctors, nurses or therapists. However, a constructive partnership between clinicians and managers is emerging as a vital component to many projects (for example, to secure the investment in service consequences discussed above). This wider view facilitates a smoother transfer of project-driven change into routine quality and service monitoring procedures

- Exploring how the approaches to *impact measurement* adopted for the project (using a basket of indicators) could be used on a continuing basis to identify when further steps may be required to reinforce the changes to clinical practice

- Ensuring that local *training and staff development programmes* are used to keep staff up to date on evidence. Induction programmes for new staff may be required.

Involving patients

An important element of all of the local project plans is to explore how patients can be involved in taking work forward on clinical effectiveness. Such involvement has implications at two main levels:

- At a broad strategic level involving the public, patients and their representatives in service planning

- At an individual level involving patients, their carers or advocates in their own care and treatment decisions.

The local project teams are involving patients in varying ways. Some project teams include patients in their teams or on the advisory group. These initiatives are aiming to use patients' views to identify needs for care and treatment, inform patient-centred progress measures and input into audit and educational activities. Various mechanisms for obtaining patients' views are being developed, including the use of focus groups or patient questionnaires.

Patients and their representatives have helped to develop patient information materials advising on their content and format. A variety of groups have been connected to the project work. These have included Community Health Councils (CHCs), voluntary organisations, patient representative groups for particular conditions and patients recruited via primary care and trusts. A range of communications channels is being used to raise public awareness about the projects and their significance for patient care, such as taking advantages of disease awareness days.

Three PACE Network discussion days focused on issues about involving patients in clinical effectiveness initiatives. Annex 6a provides notes from one of these discussions.

Evidence-based practice: a normal way of working

The initial focus of all the local projects is one particular clinical topic. The broader aim is to explore ways to translate the learning from the project to other clinical areas. Further analysis to help establish the appropriate balance of the various mechanisms for achieving change (*see* Chapter 2) may be required. For example, more time may be needed for educational activities and less time devoted to the formulation of local guidelines.

Experience so far suggests that, in the short term, someone to provide a focus for the work might be helpful (*see* Chapter 3, Lesson C2). In the longer term, better links between activities involved in managing change seem essential. Significant resources are already devoted to many of these. Better links between them could mean:

- Ensuring that clinicians have access to research evidence through local *library and information technology services*

- Assessing, through local *audit projects*, the implications of evidence and determining the need for change to local practice

- Providing appropriate *educational and development programmes*

- Ensuring arrangements are in place to *involve patients*

- Ensuring that the quality of care provided is kept under review through routine *monitoring arrangements*.

Development of these links is a task that will require a constructive partnership between clinicians and managers. It is not a challenge to be pursued solely by clinicians.

The projects are being taken forward in health authorities and NHS trusts. The challenge of making evidence-based practice a normal way of business will need to address issues from a commissioning and service provision perspective. Examples are finding the optimum way to integrate the approach into commissioning cycles and into service development plans.

Making evidence-based practice a normal way of working within organisations was the subject of the PACE discussion paper *From Project to Mainstream* (September 1996). This suggested an incremental approach – *see* Annex 5a.

Questions remain about the most effective way to manage these four aspects of work on clinical effectiveness and further consideration of these issues is planned for the second half of the PACE programme.

Chapter 6

The PACE Network

Network membership and benefits

The PACE Network provides links between people across the NHS who are interested in the promotion of evidence-based practice. The Network was launched in December 1995 and membership, which is free, offers:

- Opportunities to attend discussion days to meet other members, share experiences and problems and to learn about progress with PACE overall

- A quarterly bulletin, *Network News*, providing information about members' interests, the forthcoming programme of discussion days and notes about previous discussions

- The means to identify colleagues in other organisations with similar interests or information through the database of members' interests.

The Network has over 400 members from a wide range of organisations, although predominantly from health authorities and NHS trusts across England. Members include clinicians, managers, co-ordinators and people from academia. A wide variety of interests has been reported by members, ranging from clinical topics (such as cardiac care, wound care and learning disabilities) to broader topics (such as involving patients and organisational development). Details of members' interests are maintained on a database, which helps to facilitate the planning of the discussion days.

Discussion days

Discussion days provide opportunities for informal sharing between Network members. The open agenda and the lunch give space for participants to share the lessons from their work, discuss ideas being explored elsewhere and work through difficult current challenges, such as how to engage stakeholders or gain access to recent research evidence. The groups are kept deliberately small – a dozen or so members – to facilitate informal discussion. Attendance is free of charge, but a cancellation fee is incurred if reservations are cancelled less than ten days before the event. *Network News* is circulated to members well in advance to let them know about the future programme of discussion days.

Many Network members report that they keep in touch with other participants and inform colleagues about the days. Several have instituted new activities that follow up on ideas mentioned at the discussion days. This anecdotal expression of enthusiasm has been underlined by an evaluation of the discussion days, which reveals that:

- About 90% of participants found the discussion helpful in generating ideas for their own work

- Over 60% indicated that they were likely to keep in touch with colleagues they met at the discussion day

- About 50% indicated that they would change their approach to their work following the discussion.

Apart from members sharing ideas with like-minded individuals, the Network has provided a forum for sharing progress on the work of the 16 local PACE projects. For example, the session about back pain in June 1997 included a presentation about the project in Southern Derbyshire. Further similar presentations are planned. Members have reported that their involvement has been motivated by a desire to keep up to date with local and national developments. The open agendas and informality of the discussion days have been welcomed. The discussions have given many participants enthusiasm and confidence that they are on the right track.

Discussion topics

Between June 1996 and July 1997, 22 discussion days were arranged covering a wide range of topics (such as cardiac care, wound care and menorrhagia, and including some not covered in the local PACE projects). For example, there have been discussions about diabetes, learning disabilities, maternity services and psychology as well as some focusing on broader topics, such as patient involvement and outcomes measurement.

Some of the discussion days centred on social and community care issues and, in particular, learning disabilities, psychology and mental health. Participants in these discussions noted issues concerning the nature of evidence and that:

- The normal health model of health benefit and gain does not easily fit: there is a need to be clear about what is meant by the term 'effectiveness'

- Evidence can be sparse and diverse, with little about the effective organisation of services

- In the absence of evidence it may be useful to clarify and quantify what is being done now (current services and practice) as a starting point for change.

Often, the discussions focused on challenges in service delivery. For example, in the learning disabilities field, there were problems across primary and secondary care and particularly issues arising because people with learning disabilities are rarely in contact with primary care. The PACE team circulates notes outlining some of the main issues covered during the day as a prompt for participants. An example of these notes, following a discussion about involving patients, is in Annex 6a.

There will be more discussion days in 1998. The topic-based discussion days, some involving presentations about the local PACE projects, will be complemented by practically focused workshops, for example, about questions involved in creating clinical effectiveness strategies.

The PACE Team

The PACE programme is supported by a team based at the King's Fund. Members of the team and their contact details are:

Michael Dunning
Programme Manager
Telephone: 0171 307 2653
Email: m.dunning@kehf.org.uk

Gerrard Abi-Aad
Information and Research Officer
Telephone: 0171 307 2654
Email: g.abiaad@kehf.org.uk

David Gilbert
Project Officer
Telephone: 0171 307 2661
Email: d.gilbert@kehf.org.uk

Steve Gillam
Director, Medical Development Programme
Telephone: 0171 307 2692
Email: s.gillam@kehf.org.uk

Hayley Livett
Project Assistant
Telephone: 0171 307 2694
Email: h.livett@kehf.org.uk

The PACE team is based at:

King's Fund Development Centre
11–13 Cavendish Square
London W1M 0AN
Fax: 0171 307 2810

PACE Bulletin and Discussion Papers

A quarterly *PACE Bulletin* is circulated to all health authorities and NHS trusts:

Bulletin 1 launched the programme and described the application process.

Bulletin 2 reported on the range of applications received and launched the PACE Network.

Bulletin 3 identified the local projects selected to form the main element of the programme.

Bulletin 4 described early lessons about planning implementation projects.

Bulletin 5 described the first series of PACE discussion papers.

Bulletin 6 suggested approaches to measurement and evaluation.

Bulletin 7 described work on creating local communications strategies.

Bulletin 8 reported on discussions about working with primary care and progress in 1996.

Bulletin 9 reported on the mid-term review and links with CCEPP.

In addition, two special issues of the *PACE Bulletin* have been circulated about aspects of work on clinical effectiveness:

Involving Patients (September 1996).

Working with Primary Care (June 1997).

A series of PACE discussion papers was launched in September 1996. These are intended as concise introductions to elements of initiatives to promote clinical effectiveness:

Getting Started (September 1996) reports on a series of discussions with local PACE projects about how to go about establishing a local implementation project.

Creating Local Projects (September 1996) offers a checklist of tasks, issues and pointers to success in setting up local projects.

Measuring Impact (September 1996) describes a framework for measuring the impact of local projects.

Education, Learning and Professional Development (September 1996) offers advice about creating educational programmes to support local projects.

From Project to Mainstream (September 1996) explores issues involved in ensuring that using evidence becomes a normal way of business in organisations.

Effective Communications: the PACE experience so far (March 1997) reports on the work required to keep local staff and organisations in touch with project work. The paper draws on examples from two local PACE projects.

Implementation: the Evidence

This annex has been prepared to offer a guide to implementing clinical effectiveness. It provides a reading and resource list that may be helpful when working to secure local change. As might be expected with any rapidly developing field, this guide is not intended to provide a definitive reading list. The focus is on issues surrounding implementation – accumulating the evidence, managing change, training and education. Several texts listed report on the practical experiences of attempts to implement clinical effectiveness. They provide a valuable insight into some of the challenges involved in effecting change.

Gerrard Abi-Aad, in the PACE team, would welcome enquiries about and comments on the information given. He may be contacted at:

Telephone: 0171 307 2654
Email: g.abiaad@kehf.org.uk

Publications

Booth A. *The ScHARR guide to evidence-based practice*. ScHARR Occasional Paper No. 97/2. May 1997. The guide identifies useful sources and resources in support of evidence-based practice. In most cases only material published from 1990 onwards is included in the guide.

Eve R, Golton I, Hodgkin P, Munro J, Musson G. *Learning from FACTS – Lessons from the Framework for Appropriate Care Throughout Sheffield (FACTS) project*. ScHARR, University of Sheffield, Occasional Paper No. 97/3. May 1997. Looks at how clinical change can be brought about and describes some of the thinking and methods underpinning the work. In particular it considers motivating GPs, translating between different organisational cultures, the use of marketing techniques, the nature of development work and building coalitions of interested people to support a particular change.

Department of Health. *Methods to promote the implementation of research findings in the NHS – Priorities for evaluation*. Report to the NHS Central Research and Development Committee, October 1995. The report identifies R&D priorities on methods of transferring research into practice and describes 20 priority areas for R&D.

Dopson S E and Gabbay J. Wessex Institute of Public Health Medicine and Templeton College Oxford. *Getting Research into Practice and Purchasing – Issues and Lessons from the Four Counties*. Research commissioned by Anglia and Oxford Region, 1996. Reports on the Getting Research into Practice project in Oxford RHA (now Anglia and Oxford Region). The project explored the ways purchasers can use research evidence to inform the purchasing process. A key feature of the original project design was the importance of sharing the learning and experience across the region as the work went forward.

Dunning M, Needham G and Weston S (editors). *But Will It Work, Doctor? Report of a second 'But will it work, doctor?' conference, Northampton.* ISBN 1 898300 119. May 1996. Report of a conference about promoting and supporting patient choice by making evidence about the effectiveness of health care accessible to health service users.

Effective Health Care. Implementing clinical practice guidelines: can guidelines be used to improve clinical practice? *Effective Health Care Bulletin* No. 8. University of Leeds, Leeds, 1995.

Muir Gray J A. *Evidence-based healthcare. How to make health policy and management decisions.* Churchill Livingstone, 1997. ISBN 0 443 05721 4. The book aims to help those people who have to make decisions about groups of patients or populations base such decisions on a careful appraisal of the best evidence available.

NHS Executive. *Promoting Clinical Effectiveness – A framework for action in and through the NHS, January 1996.* This booklet is intended to help chief executives of health authorities and NHS trusts to develop ways of promoting greater clinical effectiveness throughout the NHS in primary and secondary care.

Oxman A. No magic bullets. *Canadian Medical Association Journal* 1995: 153 (10): 1423–1431. A systematic review of 102 trials of interventions to help health care professionals deliver services more effectively or efficiently.

Walshe K and Ham C. *Acting on the Evidence Progress in the NHS.* Research Paper. The University of Birmingham Health Services Management Centre, 1997. The report presents the findings of a research study that set out to assess the progress of evidence-based health care in the NHS and to identify innovations and approaches that might serve as models of good practice.

Articles

General references

Armstrong D, Reyburn H, Jones R. A study of general practitioners' reasons for changing their prescribing behaviour. *British Medical Journal* 1996; 312: 949–52.

Batstone G and Edwards M. Achieving clinical effectiveness: just another initiative or a real change in working practice? *Journal of Clinical Effectiveness* 1996; 1(1): 19–21.

Cullum N, Sheldon T. Clinically challenged. *Nursing Management* 1996; 3(4): 14–16.

Dickson R, Droogan J. Systematic reviews: examples for nursing. *Nursing Standard*. RCN Publishing Company, February 1997.

Farquhar W. Clinical effectiveness: making it happen. *Audit Trends* 1996; 4 (3): 85.

Graham G. Clinical effectiveness in a rational health service: strategic partnerships can make it a reality. *Health Director* 1996; Jun (22): 11–12.

Haines A, Jones R. Implementing findings of research. *British Medical Journal* 1994; 308: 1488–92.

MacDonald J. Opportunity or threat? *IHSM Network* 1996; Mar 3 (6): 5–6.

Murphy M, Dunning M. Implementing clinical effectiveness – is it time for a change of gear? *British Journal of Health Care Management* 1997; 3 (1): 23–26.

Sackett D L, Rosenberg W M C, Gray J A M, Haynes R B, Richardson W S. Evidence based medicine: what it is and what it isn't. *British Medical Journal* 1996; 312: 71–72.

References related to education and training

Davis D A. *The dissemination of information: Optimising the effectiveness of continuing medical education. Disseminating research/changing practice. Research methods for primary care.* Vol 6, Chapter III. Sage 1994: 139–50.

Elliot P, Pickering S. The purpose of PREP. *Nursing management (UK)* 1997; 4(3): 12–13.

Muir Gray J A. Evidence-based public health: what level of competence is required? *Journal of Public Health Medicine* 1997; 19(1): 65–68.

Normand C. Professionals in the NHS. *British Journal of Healthcare Management* 1997; 3(5): 280–81.

Pearson P, Jones K. Developing professional knowledge: making primary care education and research more relevant. *BMJ* 1997; 314(7083): 817–820.

Wright S, Gough P, Mortlock R. The future of nurse education. *Nursing Standard* 1997; 11(34): 22–27.

Contacts list

Cochrane Collaboration on Effective Professional Practice (CCEPP)

CCEPP undertakes reviews of interventions designed to improve health professionals' practice and delivery of health services. This includes educational, behavioural, organisational, financial and regulatory interventions. CCEPP reviews can be found in the Cochrane Library.

Contact:

Graham Mowatt
CCEPP, Health Services Research Unit, Department of Public Health,
Polwarth Building, Drew Kay Wing, Forester Hill, Aberdeen AB25 2ZD
Tel: 01224 681818 ext 51100
Fax: 01224 663087
Email: ccepp@abdn.ac.uk

Critical Appraisal Skills Programme (CASP)

A training service to help health service decision makers develop skills in the critical appraisal of evidence about effectiveness, in order to promote the delivery of evidence-based health care.

Contact:

Claire Spittlehouse
Critical Appraisal Skills Programme, Institute of Health Sciences,
Anglia and Oxford RHA, Old Road, Headington, Oxford OX3 7LF
Tel: 01865 226968
Fax: 01865 226775

Health Care Evaluation Unit (HCEU)

HCEU is a designated support unit for the National Research and Development Initiative (South Thames) located within the Department of Public Health Sciences at St George's Hospital Medical School. The unit has recently developed an instrument for assessing the quality of clinical guidelines and has been appointed by the DoH to quality assure nationally developed guidelines.

Contact:

Dr Peter Littlejohns
Health Care Evaluation Unit
Dept. of Public Health Sciences
St George's Hospital Medical School
Crammer Terrace
Tooting
London
SW17 0RE
Tel: 0181 725 5419/28
Fax: 0181 725 3584

National Centre for Clinical Audit (NCCA)

The centre has been established to:

● create a national clinical audit information and dissemination centre

- encourage participation in, and improve the quality of, multi-disciplinary audit through sharing the principles of effective audit and examples of good audit practice

- develop criteria for excellence in clinical audit and develop a national database of clinical audits.

Contact:

Dr Mark Charny
National Centre for Clinical Audit
BMA House
Tavistock Square
London
WC1H 9JP
Tel: 0171 383 6451
Fax: 0171 383 6373
Email: NCCA@kcl.ac.uk

NHS Executive Clinical Effectiveness Reference Pack

This reference pack, available since October 1996, contains documents that provide reference material to those involved in promoting clinical effectiveness in the NHS.

Useful Web sites

Bandolier

Bandolier is a monthly evidence-based medicine journal produced in Oxford for the NHS R&D Directorate. It contains bullet points of evidence-based medicine, hence its title. The editors are Andrew Moore, with Henry McQuay and Muir Gray. *Bandolier* Internet access is free, but it may run several months behind the printed version. Subscription to the printed version of *Bandolier* costs £30 per year (UK) and £60 overseas (subscriptions and back numbers).

http: //www.jr2.ox.ac.uk: 80/bandolier/

Centre for Evidence-Based Medicine

The Centre for Evidence-Based Medicine in Oxford aims to promote evidence-based health care and provide support and resources.

http: //cebm.jr2.ox.ac.uk

Centre for Reviews and Dissemination

The NHS Centre for Reviews and Dissemination (CRD) in York aims to identify and review the results of good quality health research and to disseminate the findings to key decision makers in the NHS and to consumers of health care services. The reviews cover the effectiveness of care for particular conditions, the effectiveness of health technologies and evidence on efficient methods of organising and delivering particular types of health care.

http: //www.york.ac.uk/inst/crd/welcome.htm

Cochrane Collaboration

Provides access to information on all Cochrane activities and to the Cochrane handbook. There is also password-protected access to some of the reviews.

http: //hiru.mcmaster.ca/COCHRANE/DEFAULT.htm

Critical Appraisal Skills Programme

A resource for health service decision makers and those who seek to influence decision makers – to help them develop skills in the critical appraisal of evidence about effectiveness, in order to promote the delivery of evidence-based health care.

http: //www.ihs.ox.ac.uk/casp/

Health Technology Assessment

Health Technology Assessment is the largest single programme of work within the NHS R&D Programme. It takes a broad view of the term 'Health Technology' covering all interventions, including the use of devices, equipment, drugs, procedures and care across the whole spectrum of medical, nursing and health practices. The programme aims to address the questions of purchasers, providers and users of health services on the effectiveness and cost-effectiveness of interventions. Does this treatment work? For whom? At what cost? How does it compare to other treatments that are available?

http: //www.wiphm.soton.ac.uk/hta/ *but moving to* http: //www.soton.ac.uk/~wi/hta

ScHARR

The School of Health and Related Research (ScHARR, pronounced shah) was formed in 1994 to act as a focus for health services research/health technology assessment within the University of Sheffield. ScHARR harnesses the strengths of a number of methodological teams, including expertise in health services management, health services research, health economics, information science, operational research and statistics and conducts research in a broad variety of clinical settings, including ageing, general practice, nursing, rehabilitation, mental health and public health.

http: //www.shef.ac.uk/uni/academic/R-Z/scharr/

PACE Local Projects

This annex provides details of the individual local projects, giving:

- A brief pen-picture of each project
- The evidence that provides the basis for the work
- A note of locally produced material (there might be a modest charge to cover printing and postage)
- Contact details for the project leader.

The 16 local PACE projects are:

1. Barnet Health Authority – Hypertension

2. Bradford Health Authority – *Helicobacter pylori* eradication

3. Bromley – *Helicobacter pylori* eradication

4. Chase Farm Hospitals NHS Trust – Pressure sores

5. Dorset Health Authority – Menorrhagia

6. Dudley Health Authority – Continence

7. Gloucestershire Royal NHS Trust – The management of stroke patients

8. Lambeth, Southwark and Lewisham Health Authority and King's Health Care – Cardiac rehabilitation

9. North Derbyshire Health Authority – Congestive cardiac failure

10. Oxfordshire Health Authority – Post-operative pain control

11. Royal Berkshire and Battle Hospitals NHS Trust – Leg ulcers

12. South Tyneside Health Care Trust – Stable angina

13. Southern Derbyshire – Low back pain

14. Walsall Health Authority – *Helicobacter pylori* eradication

15. Wigan and Bolton Health Authority – Continence

16. Wirral Health Authority – Family support in schizophrenia

1. Barnet Health Authority – Hypertension

This project is developing a collaborative approach for stroke prevention by providing evidence-based information on effective interventions to primary care teams. Another key feature is the development of a programme of professional education for GPs and practice nurses. Other professions included in the programme are pharmacists, health promotion specialists and local stroke association volunteers.

Screening of all Barnet residents over 60 for modifiable stroke risk factors has been encouraged. The health authority is also promoting the development of hypertension registers and the use of patient education and patient-held records. Audit will be used to monitor the implementation of stroke risk factor management.

The evidence

Using the evidence: Northamptonshire project on stroke. Stroke literature review. Northamptonshire Health Authority. 1994.

Wolfe *et al. Stroke services and research.* The Stroke Association 1996.

Collins *et al.* Benefits of lowering BP in the general population: review of 14 randomised trials of antihypertensives. *Lancet* 1990; 335: 827–38.

Sanderson S. Hypertension in the elderly: pressure to treat? *Health Trends* 1996; 28(4).

Local material

The following items are available from the local project leader:

● Handout summarising evidence on hypertension and discussing proposed audit
● Pilot audit tool
● Hypertension guideline (draft)
● Patient record and information leaflet (draft)
● Education and presentation pack (draft).

Project leader

Dr Tony Isaacs
Consultant in Clinical Audit, Education and Training
Barnet Health Authority, Department of Public Health,
Hyde House, The Hyde, Edgware Road, London NW9 6QQ
Tel: 0181 201 4700
Fax: 0181 201 4702

The project co-ordinator, Ms Julie Gottlieb, can be contacted at the same address.

2. Bradford Health Authority – *Helicobacter pylori* eradication

This project is developing a co-ordinated evidence-based approach to the management of dyspepsia, in particular to ensure that patients with known duodenal ulcer on repeat H_2 antagonists receive eradication therapy for *H. pylori*. This is in line with research evidence that *H. pylori* eradication can cure duodenal ulcers.

Key tasks are to produce and implement local evidence-based clinical guidelines on the management of dyspepsia that are integrated into referral forms and computer protocols and to conduct audits across primary and secondary care based on routinely available data.

A re-audit of practice aims to assess the proportion of patients going on to receive eradication therapy. Other baseline measures that will provide progress measures are the numbers of endoscopies carried out, the appropriateness of referrals for endoscopy, changes in requests for breath tests and *H. pylori* serology tests and alterations in prescribing.

The evidence

Evidence for clinical guidelines collated from a systematic review of the literature and critical appraisal (list of references available on request).

Evidence for the implementation methods was obtained from the Cochrane Collaboration for Effective Clinical Practice.

Local material

The following items are available from the local project leader:

- Evidence-based guidelines for the management of patients with dyspepsia
- Evidence-based guidelines for the management of patients' post-endoscopy
- Endoscopy referral form with integrated guideline
- Summary of methodology and group members involved in guideline development
- Patient information leaflet and booklet.

Project leader

Dr John Wright
Consultant Epidemiologist
Bradford Royal Infirmary,
Duckworth Lane,
Bradford BD9 6RJ
Tel: 01274 364279
Fax: 01274 364026

Project manager

Ms Julie Hughes
Bradford Health Authority
New Mill,
Victoria Road,
Saltaire, Shipley, BD18 3LD
Tel: 01274 366032

3. Bromley – *Helicobacter pylori* eradication

The focus for this joint health authority and local hospital project is the treatment of patients with proven ulcers who are on long-term drug treatments. This topic was chosen because as well as being of interest to local clinicians, the evidence for change was clear (the eradication of *H. pylori*) and change should secure significant health care benefits. From the outset participation by primary care practitioners was regarded as essential. Initially the work is being taken forward with six practices, chosen to be broadly representative in terms of practice population size and ulcer-related prescribing.

There are two aspects to the work. First, an educational approach based on small group discussions and practical examples to explore the benefits of change for practices and patients. These sessions also engage GPs in the use of evidence in developing guidelines and reviewing current practice. Second, the local project team is working with practices to identify patients whose current treatment appears to merit review. The intention is to use the experience from the work with the pilot practices to develop a programme to include all practices in Bromley.

The evidence

Moore R A. *Helicobacter pylori and peptic ulcer: a systematic review of effectiveness and an overview of the economic benefits of implementing what is known to be effective.* Health Technology and Evaluation Association. Oxford. 1995.

Penston J G. Review article: Helicobacter pylori eradication – understandable caution but no excuse for inertia. *Alimentary Pharmacology and Therapeutics.* 1994; 8(4): 369–89.

Powell K U *et al.* Helicobacter pylori eradication in patients with peptic ulcer disease: clinical consequences and financial implications. *Qtly Jnl Med* 1994; 87: 283–90.

Local material

The following items are available from the local project leader:

- Case study scenarios
- Education and evidence packs for 3 areas: Who to Treat, How to Test, How to Treat
- Current draft guidelines
- Draft operational guide for conducting audit to identify proven ulcer disease patients
- Pack showing the implications of identifying and changing treatments for proven ulcer disease
- Draft contract for pharmaceutical company involvement.

Project leader

Mr Steve Dewar
Head of Bromley Applied Research Unit
Bromley Hospitals NHS Trust, Elmswood Building, Farnborough Hospital,
Farnborough Common, Orpington, Kent BR6 8ND
Tel: 01689 814377; Fax: 01689 862423

4. Chase Farm Hospitals NHS Trust – Pressure sores

This project seeks to reduce the incidence of hospital-acquired pressure sores and improve the management of existing pressure sores. The work is co-ordinated by a small core project group involving a range of disciplines, including managers, clinicians and therapists, but also the surgical appliances officer and the porters, who need to move equipment. Key tasks include: improving data collection, developing local evidence-based guidelines and establishing audit procedures on pressure care and wound management. An educational programme has been introduced and a local wound care group, which includes link nurses for each clinical area, helps to disseminate information and review products relating to wound care and pressure sore prevention. To spread the message, local communication channels are being utilised, including the medical audit group and practice management group meetings. Outcome measures include changes in the number of hospital-acquired pressure sores.

The evidence

Effective Health Care. *The prevention and treatment of pressure sores.* Universities of Leeds and York. NHS Centre for Reviews and Dissemination. 1995; 2(1): 1–16.

Effective Health Care. *Implementing clinical practice guidelines.* Universities of Leeds and York. NHS Centre for Reviews and Dissemination. 1994; 1(8): 1–11.

McNaughton V, Brazil K. Impact of education on pressure sore prevalence in chronic care. *Journal of Gerontological Nursing* 1995; 21(2): 45–49.

Local material

The following items are available from the local project leader:

- Pressure Care and Wound Care Resource File (good practice guidelines)
- Wound assessment tool
- Pressure sore incidence data collection form
- Mattress audit tool
- Dressing evaluation report.

Project leader

Ms Janice Sigsworth
Director of Nursing, Chase Farm Hospitals NHS Trust,
The Ridgeway, Enfield, Middlesex EN2 8JL
Tel: 0181 366 6600
Fax: 0181 366 1361

The project co-ordinator, Ms Julie Baker, can be contacted at the same address.

5. Dorset Health Authority – Menorrhagia

This project aims to improve the diagnosis and medical and surgical management of menorrhagia across primary and secondary care. There is national evidence of excessive numbers of D&Cs and hysterectomies performed on women suffering from menorrhagia and inappropriate prescribing of hormonal treatments. The main objectives of the project are to reduce the number of D&Cs performed and to alter prescribing patterns towards more effective drug treatments.

There are five main tasks being undertaken. First, to develop and implement evidence-based clinical guidelines on the management of menorrhagia – a standard referral letter has been designed that is included in the GP guidelines. Second, to disseminate these via existing communications channels, such as the Trust Clinical Effectiveness and Audit Committees and through educational programmes for GPs, pharmacists, hospital medical and nursing staff throughout Dorset. Third, to re-audit practice across primary and secondary care and establish compliance with the guidelines. Fourth, to involve patients in the production of appropriate information materials. Fifth, to develop fast-track, one-stop diagnostic clinics for menorrhagia in each of the local acute trusts.

The evidence

Effective Health Care Bulletin. Management of Menorrhagia, Aug 95 (*see* reference list contained in Bulletin).

Local material

The following items are available from the local project leader:

- Briefing document for June 1996 steering group
- Leaflet explaining the Dorset menorrhagia project
- Draft secondary care guidelines
- CHC menorrhagia recruitment leaflet
- CHC questionnaire for women suffering from menorrhagia
- Sources of evidence on effective clinical practice in managing menorrhagia
- Set of three GP questionnaires
- Guidelines for the management of abnormal vaginal bleeding.

Project leader

Dr Vicky Hempsall
Deputy Director of Public Health, Dorset Health Authority,
Victoria House, Princes Road, Ferndown, Dorset BH22 9JR
Tel: 01202 893000
Fax: 01202 861125

The project manager, Ms Joy Reynolds, can be contacted at the same address.

6. Dudley Health Authority – Continence

This project focuses on urinary incontinence – in particular, to alleviate the distress suffered from this condition by women under 65. A multi-disciplinary strategy at primary and secondary care level is being developed for the promotion of continence and management of incontinence. The three areas of the strategy are: raising awareness among public and professionals, improving preventive measures and making effective treatment more accessible. Underlying this is the major theme of training nurses to screen women so that those with simple stress incontinence can be managed by nurses, while more complex problems can be referred to the continence advisory service.

Support for professionals includes educational seminars and the circulation of a continence products directory. For the public, awareness-raising events complement the development of patient information leaflets. Progress measures based on routinely available data have included numbers and type of operative procedures for incontinence, referrals to the continence advisory service and expenditure on incontinence pads and other aids and appliances.

The evidence

Agency for Health Care Policy and Research. *Urinary incontinence in adults: clinical practice guidelines*. Pub No 92-0038: US Dept Health and Human Services, Rockville, MD, 1992.

Royal College of Physicians. *Incontinence: causes, management and provision of services*. London: RCP, 1995.

Brocklehurst N. *Purchasing for continence promotion: guidelines for health authorities and GP fundholders on commissioning continence services*. West Midlands Regional Health Authority, 1994.

Local material

The following items are available from the local project leader:

- Training pack for practice nurses, including patient assessment pro formas
- Pelvic floor exercise leaflet (with translations in seven community languages)
- An information leaflet on urinary incontinence in nursing and residential homes.

Project leader

Dr Alison Hamilton
Director of Public Health, Dudley Health,
12 Bull Street, Dudley DY1 2DD
Tel: 01384 239376
Fax: 01384 455068

The project manager, Dr Wendy Phillips, can be contacted at the same address.

7. Gloucestershire Royal NHS Trust – The management of stroke patients

This trust-led project focuses on stroke care. The evidence shows that specialist stroke multi-disciplinary teams enhance the effectiveness of post-stroke care. With this in mind, the project team are developing an 'integrated care pathway' (ICP) for acute care and rehabilitation drawing together different professional assessment procedures and acting as the focus for multi-disciplinary working. A staff training programme helped to explain the ICP and treatment and care needs of patients and carers. The reorganisation of services has resulted in a streamlined referral process and designated stroke beds.

Outcome measures include assessing variations from the ICP and measuring the project's impact on length of stay and costs. Lessons from the work are being shared internally and externally, for example, to the trust board, CHC and local councillors. The ICP for stroke also provides a useful template for work in other diagnoses, and ICPs are being developed in all clinical specialities. Early ICPs include nephrectomy, abdominal aortic aneurysm and myocardial infarction.

The evidence

Kaira L *et al.* Improving stroke rehabilitation. A controlled study. *Stroke* 1994; 25(4): 911–12.

Warlow C *et al.* Stroke Unit Trialists' Collaboration. *A systematic review of specialist multidisciplinary (stroke unit) care for stroke inpatients.* Stroke module of the Cochrane database of systematic reviews. London BMJ Publishing Group. 1995.

Goodyear H M. Can admission notes be improved by using pre-printed assessment sheets? *Quality in Health Care* 1995; 4: 190–93.

Local material

The following items are available from the local project leader:

- Clerking pro forma (based on material developed by the Royal College of Physicians), which forms the basis of medical documentation in the care pathway
- Nursing assessment form (adapted and developed from Barthel Activities of Daily Living Scale)
- Data sheet to support data collection and benchmarking (through the European Stroke Database and Co-star based in Newcastle)
- Reference source of evidence-based care.

Project leader

Ms Janet Duberley
Nursing Executive Director,
Gloucestershire Royal NHS Trust, Great Western Road, Gloucester GL1 3NN
Tel: 01452 394666; Fax: 01452 394737

The project manager, Ms Bev Williams, can be contacted in the Dept of Clinical Audit, at the same address.

8. Lambeth, Southwark and Lewisham Health Authority and King's Health Care – Cardiac rehabilitation

This project is embedded within a wider clinical effectiveness programme at the health authority. It focuses on developing a cardiac rehabilitation service at primary and secondary care level. This is in order to increase uptake of rehabilitation programmes by patients and their families and ensure a smooth transition from secondary to primary and community care.

Developing and implementing local evidence-based guidelines is complemented by four main activities. First, developmental work with local primary care practices supporting effective cardiac intervention throughout the primary health care team. Second, working with small groups of patients, a method has been developed to teach primary health care teams effective management from the patient's point of view. Third, the development of proxy outcomes for evaluation. Fourth, a dissemination strategy uses existing communications channels across local organisations, including the health promotion agency Health First.

The evidence

Oldbridge N B et al. Cardiac rehabilitation after myocardial infarction: combined experience of randomised controlled clinical trials. JAMA 1988; 260: 945–50.

Horgen J et al. Working party report on cardiac rehabilitation. Br Heart J 1992; 67: 412–18.

Wilhelmsson C et al. Smoking and myocardial infarction. Lancet 1975; 302: 415–20.

Randomised trial of cholesterol lowering in 4444 patients with coronary heart disease: the Scandinavian Simvastatin Survival Study (4S). Lancet 1994; 344: 1383–89.

Local material

The following items are available from the local project leader:

- Aspirin leaflet
- Implementing Clinical Effectiveness (ICE) guidelines
- General description of PACE project
- Training pack for practice and district nurses in ischaemic heart disease
- Audit pack produced by local Medical Audit Advisory Group (MAAG)
- ICE guidelines translated into lay language.

Project leader

Dr Brian Fisher
Primary Care Development Practitioner,
Lambeth, Southwark and Lewisham Health Authority,
1 Lower Marsh, London SE1 7NT
Tel: 0171 716 7000
Fax: 0171 716 7018

9. North Derbyshire Health Authority – Congestive cardiac failure

The focus of this project is on improving the investigation and management of patients with congestive heart failure. Key objectives are to increase the prescribing of ACE inhibitors and the development of open-access echocardiography. An important stimulus for the project was that local GPs were concerned about standards of care.

Work is being taken forward in three areas. First, to support GPs to undertake audit of their current practice and identify patients whose current treatment may merit review (practices representing about 90% of the population have joined in – a good indication of the scale of interest). Second, to provide an educational programme about congestive heart failure. GPs and primary health care teams have been offered a range of locality and practice-based sessions. All of these award PGEA accreditation. The emphasis is on information about the condition and treatment, not on the rigid application of strict guidelines. Third, to secure improved access to diagnostic echocardiography in the five acute hospitals providing services for local patients. One element of this service is the temporary provision of a mobile echo machine that was loaned by a pharmaceutical company to bridge a gap until a hospital-based service becomes available.

The evidence

Garg R, Yusuf S. ACE collaboration group. JAMA 1995; 273(18): 1450–56.

Rector T S. ACE inhibitors and quality of life. *Coronary Artery Disease* 1995; 6(4): 310–14.

Davie A P, McMurray J J. Economics/cost-effectiveness of ACE inhibitors. *Coronary Artery Disease* 1995; 6(4): 315–19.

Francis C M *et al*. Open access echocardiography in management of heart failure in the community. *British Medical Journal* 1995; 310: 634–36.

Local material

The following items are available from the local project leader:

- Audit pro forma
- Quality of life questionnaires
- Practice information pack
- Summary of research evidence
- Patient information leaflet

Project leader

Dr Carol Singleton
Consultant in Public Health, North Derbyshire Health,
Scarsdale, Newbold Road, Chesterfield, S41 7PF
Tel: 01246 231255
Fax: 01246 277919

The project officer, Ms Anne Hayes, can be contacted at the same address.

10. Oxfordshire Health Authority – Post-operative pain control

This project involves the health authority, a teaching hospital (the Oxford Radcliffe NHS Trust) and a district general hospital (Horton General Hospital NHS Trust) in improving the care of patients suffering from post-operative pain. It seeks to compare the differences between promoting evidence-based pain management in a teaching hospital and district general hospital and to promote trust-wide policies on acute pain management. It also aims to develop evidence-based guidelines and to implement them via a comprehensive educational and training programme. Project activities include collecting baseline data via patient questionnaires regarding severity of pain, and developing professional protocols for pain management and patient information materials.

The evidence

Royal College of Surgeons of England, Royal College of Anaesthetists. *Report of the working party on pain after surgery*. London, Royal College of Surgeons 1990.

Agency for Health Care Policy and Research. *Acute pain management in adults: operative procedures. Quick Reference Guide for Clinicians*. AHCPR Pub No. 92-0019, US Dept of Health and Human Services, Rockville, MD, 1992 (updated 1994).

Gould TH *et al*. Policy for controlling pain after surgery: effects of sequential changing in management. *British Medical Journal* 1992; 305: 1187–93.

Local material

The following items are available from the local project leader:

Handbooks: An introduction to acute pain management; a guide to patient-controlled analgesia (for the two hospitals).

Information leaflets: Post-operative pain assessment and observation chart (for the two hospitals); guidelines for intra-muscular analgesia (including treatment algorithm); guidelines for patient-controlled analgesia (in adults); guidelines for epidural analgesia (for nurses); epidural infusion algorithm for pain relief after abdominal procedures (for nurses); protocol for the management of respiratory depression (for nurses and doctors); treatment of adult post-operative nausea and vomiting (for nurses and doctors); guide to patient-controlled analgesia (for patients); pain relief after your operation (for patients, adapted with grateful permission from the Queen's Medical Centre, Nottingham).

Nursing care plans: Nursing care plan for patient controlled analgesia; nursing care plan for intra-muscular analgesia.

Questionnaires: Post-operative acute pain assessment questionnaire (adapted from the widely used Cardiff questionnaire, as used by the DoH); post-operative pain at home: a questionnaire for self-completion by recently discharged patients.

Project leader

Dr Nicholas Hicks
Consultant Public Health Physician, Oxfordshire Health Authority,
Department of Public Health and Health Policy, Old Road, Headington,
Oxford OX3 7LG
Tel: 01865 226578; Fax: 01865 226894

11. Royal Berkshire and Battle Hospitals NHS Trust – Leg ulcers

This joint venture between the local acute and community trusts focuses on improved management of leg ulcers. The project objectives are to rationalise treatment regimens, reduce variations in treatment of leg ulcers in order to accelerate healing, alleviate associated pain and reduce duration and cost of treatment. Building on an established multi-professional tissue viability group, which includes health authority representation, four working sub-groups have been established to focus on key development areas.

First, a clinical audit group is designing and piloting an audit record and supports the collection of baseline data. Second, an assessment and protocol group is developing an evidence-based assessment tool and treatment protocols. Third, a staff education group is implementing a clinician educational programme for hospital and community staff. Fourth, a patient involvement group is to record patient experiences and develop information material. A communications strategy builds on many locally produced newsletters and formal and informal groups, including newsletters to GPs, managers and clinical directors and the Community Health Council (CHC).

The evidence

Douglas W S, Simpson N B. Guidelines for the management of chronic venous leg ulceration: Report of the multidisciplinary workshop. *British Journal of Dermatology* 1995; 132: 446–52.

Callum M J *et al.* Lothian and Forth Valley leg ulcer healing trial pt1: Elastic vs non elastic bandaging in the treatment of chronic leg ulceration. *Phlebology* 1992; 7: 136–41.

Fletcher A, Cullum N, Sheldon T A. A systematic review of compression treatment for venous leg ulcers. *British Medical Journal* 1997; 315: 576–80.

Local material

The following items are available from the local project leader:

- Audit report
- Economic assessment
- Local communications strategy.

Project leader

Ms Chrissy Dunn
Senior Nurse Practice Development, Royal Berkshire and Battle Hospitals NHS Trust, Battle Hospital, Oxford Road, Reading RG3 1AG
Tel: 01734 583666 ext 6508
Fax: 01734 636438

12. South Tyneside Health Care Trust – Stable angina

This project is implementing evidence-based guidelines for chronic stable angina in primary and secondary care via therapeutic, investigative and risk factor management. Audit activities in approximately 30 general practices are accompanied by the production of a guideline pack. The pack incorporates a laminated form of the guidelines, explanation of the evidence and pertinent information sheets. These are being disseminated widely. Other main elements of the programme include an education programme for practice nurses, managers' forums, trust staff, GPs and community pharmacists. This educational programme serves as a model for the introduction of evidence-based practice. The involvement of patients through focus groups and the development of a patient-held record is viewed as a lever to help stimulate clinical change.

The evidence

North of England stable angina guideline development group. North of England evidence based guidelines development project: summary version of evidence based guideline for the primary care management of stable angina. *BMJ* 1994; 312: 827–32.

Antiplatelet Trialist Collaboration. Collaborative overview of randomised trials of antiplatelet therapy in prevention of death, myocardial infarction and stroke by prolonged antiplatelet therapy in various categories of patients. *BMJ* 1994; 308: 81–106.

Yusuf S *et al*. Beta blockage during and after myocardial infarction. An overview of the randomised trials. *Prog Cardiovasc Dis* 1985; 27: 335–71.

Local material

The following items are available from the local project leader:

A guidelines pack including: The angina guidelines; an explanation of their functions and the development process; the consensus guidelines from the British Hypertension Society on the management of hypertension; a local protocol for managing hyperlipidaemia; a drug explanation sheet; an information sheet on exercise ECGs and their function; a list of local contacts; an explanation of and relationships with other projects such as Heart Save and FACTS; an explanation of other district cardiac initiatives.

Also available are: a draft patient-held record; the publicity poster and leaflet; the education programme (needs assessment tool, programme outline and evaluation tool); a study guide; educational display boards.

Project leader

Dr John Parr
Consultant Physician, South Tyneside Health Care Trust,
South Tyneside District Hospital, Harton Lane, South Shields,
Tyne and Wear NE34 0PL
Tel: 0191 454 8888
Fax: 0191 202 4180

13. Southern Derbyshire – Low back pain

This project aims to provide improved care and treatment for people suffering acute back pain. The evidence shows that many patients with acute back pain need prompt referral to physical therapies (physiotherapy, osteopathy, chiropractic), should be encouraged to stay as active as possible and should receive more than just symptomatic pain relief. In translating the evidence into practice, the health authority also recognised a groundswell of GP opinion that there were local problems, such as excessive waiting times for physiotherapy.

Local trusts are being encouraged to prioritise patients with acute back pain problems where there is good evidence for effective interventions. This also means improving the co-ordination of specialist services and developing and implementing evidence-based guidelines. A standardised referral form is being piloted, which allows physiotherapists to identify whether a referral has been appropriate. GPs' inappropriate use of plain lumbar spine X-rays is being monitored, alongside assessment of surgical interventions and frequency of physiotherapy contact. The project team are disseminating the lessons from their work, training and educating health professionals and raising public awareness of back pain treatment.

The evidence

Clinical Standards Advisory Group – *Back Pain*. 1995.

Waddell G *et al*. *Low back pain evidence review*. Royal College of General Practitioners. 1996.

Local material

The following items are available from the local project leader:

- Guidelines for the management of acute back pain in primary care
- Back pain leaflet
- Evaluation of the Southern Derbyshire Back Pain PACE Project – Baseline Study. Newbronner L, Klaber-Moffet J, Croucher K, Place M, University of York/York Health Economics Consortium
- Physiotherapy audit tool
- Report of a Search Conference on People's Experience of Back Pain. Spear S P, Southern Derbyshire Health
- Clinical guidelines in Southern Derbyshire – guideline development pack.

Project leader

Dr Steve Whitehead
Director of Public Health, South Derbyshire Health,
Derwent Court, Stuart Street, Derby DE1 2FZ
Tel: 01332 626300; Fax: 01332 626350

The project manager, Mr Steve Spear, can be contacted at the same address.

14. Walsall Health Authority – *Helicobacter pylori* eradication

This project aims to implement a disease management programme for dyspepsia, concentrating on *H. pylori* eradication in existing patients with peptic ulcer disease, and developing a consistent and rational approach to managing dyspepsia. In particular, the intention is to develop local guidance on upper gastrointestinal disease across primary and secondary care and promote the guidelines in partnership with the local gastroenterologists, GP educators, audit groups and Keele University. Main activities include: setting up procedures for the collection and analysis of data, developing monitoring systems, identifying potential cases via local primary care practices, promoting practice nurse training and developing information for GPs and patients.

The evidence

Moore R A. *Helicobacter pylori and peptic ulcer: a systematic review of effectiveness and an overview of the economic benefits of implementing what is known to be effective.* Health Technology and Evaluation Association. Oxford. 1995.

National Institutes of Health Consensus Conference. *Helicobacter pylori in peptic ulcer disease.* NIH Consensus Statement. 1994.

Helicobacter pylori and peptic ulcer. Centre for Reviews and Dissemination. *Effectiveness Matters* 1995; 1: issue 2.

Local material

The following items are available from the local project leader:

- Clinical management pathway for the management of dyspepsia
- Data collection form for a specialist GI nurse or PHC nurse
- Information for GPs – evidence to support the pathway
- Open access endoscopy audit form for administration by nurse during pre-investigation clerking
- New hospital referral form for upper GI endoscopy
- Patient information booklet
- Case finding pro forma for practice staff
- Revised open access endoscopy form.

Project leader

Dr Jeff Norwood
Consultant in Public Health Medicine,
Walsall Health, 27–31 Lichfield House, Walsall, S1 1TE
Tel: 01922 720255
Fax: 01922 722051

15. Wigan and Bolton Health Authority – Continence

This project is helping to improve district-wide continence services, in particular by implementing research evidence indicating that incontinence can be cured or improved if accurately assessed and managed appropriately. The implementation of guidelines that include referral and assessment is complemented by an educational programme for professionals, users and carers.

Evaluation of the use of a locally developed continence assessment and referral form is one of a number of assessment measures. Others include:

- Assessment of number and type of referrals to secondary care for urinary incontinence
- Management of those already in receipt of continence materials
- In-patient gynaecology activity for incontinence
- Waiting times for physiotherapy
- Prescribing patterns
- Consumer audit.

The evidence

Royal College of Physicians. *Incontinence: causes, management and provision of services. Report of a working party.* London. 1995.

Agency of Health Care Policy and Research. *Urinary incontinence in adults: clinical practice guideline.* AHCPR. US Department of Health and Human Services. Rockville. USA. 1992.

Local material

The following items are available from the local project leader:

- Guidelines for the management of adult urinary incontinence
- Information to support the guidelines
- Assessment and referral forms for urinary incontinence in primary care
- Treatment plans
- Patient information booklet
- Information booklet for GPs about the Continence Advisory Service.

Project leader

Dr Sally Bradley
Medical Director, Community Healthcare Bolton,
St Peter's House, Silverwell Street, Bolton BL1 1PP
Tel: 01204 377000
Fax: 01204 377004

16. Wirral Health Authority – Family support in schizophrenia

This partnership involving the health authority, the voluntary organisation Making Space, the community trust, social services and a local mental health forum aims to improve the care of those suffering from schizophrenia. Evidence suggests that psycho-social interventions aimed at supporting families where there is a sufferer of schizophrenia can reduce hospital admissions and relapse and ease the burden on families. To put this research evidence into practice, a family support worker (FSW) has been employed to work within a multi-disciplinary team. The FSW has an active case-load of approximately 30 families, with other families being supported by a newly developed carers group.

The project will assess the impact on families and the team itself, as well as looking at the strategic consequences of this type of team working. The project has involved a gradual introduction of the service, originally to six GP practice populations and after almost a year expanded to 20 practices. Issues that have required careful handling to date include confidentiality and the integration of non-NHS staff into an NHS team.

The evidence

Mari J J, Steiner D. Family intervention for those with schizophrenia. *Cochrane Library* 1996; Issue 2.

Huxley P. Making More Space: *The unique and vital contribution of the family support worker*. University of Manchester, 1994.

Local material

The following items are available from the local project leader:

- Objectives for the project from the point of view of the key stakeholders (health authority, Making Space and the Department of Psychiatry)
- Notes from a workshop to discuss the role of the FSW and lessons for the development of community mental health teams
- Project communications network.

Project leader

Mr Nick Morris
Commissioning Manager,
Wirral Health Authority, St Catherine's Hospital, Clock Tower, Church Road,
Tranmere, Birkenhead L42 0LQ
Tel: 0151 651 0011
Fax: 0151 652 2668

Barriers to Change

During the early phase of setting up the local projects, discussions with some of the project leaders identified the following points as possible barriers that would have to be overcome as the work was taken forward. These notes formed part of the PACE discussion paper *Getting Started* (September 1996).

Lack of perception of relevance

Even if people are aware of the clinical effectiveness agenda, they are unlikely to have critically appraised their own practice, or they may feel that they are already working in a clinically effective manner.

Lack of resources

Setting up a clinical effectiveness project is a resource-intensive exercise and many health professionals may feel that they do not have the time or money to become involved.

Short-term outlook

Achieving change must be seen as a long-term issue. This does not sit well with annual contracting circles. Projects must be developed alongside the commissioning and contracting cycles.

Conflicting priorities

This may be particularly relevant when trying to secure senior commitment. Other local management priorities – such as the waiting list initiative – may conflict with achieving effective care.

The difficulty in measuring outcomes

It may not be understood that, because the topic has already been shown to be effective, outcomes do not need to be demonstrated. What needs to be demonstrated is the effective implementation of the project. This can be achieved using routinely available process measures.

Lack of necessary skills

Unfamiliar skills are needed, such as critical appraisal of the research literature and communication skills.

No history of multi-disciplinary working

It is very likely that the project will span clinical disciplines. Often, members of different disciplines are not used to working together in a collaborative fashion.

Limitations of the research evidence on effectiveness

The clinical effectiveness agenda may be viewed with scepticism by health professionals. Criticisms cited include the fact that available evidence often has limited applicability, clinical freedom may be lost, and services may be cut in the name of clinical effectiveness.

Perverse incentives

These may exert pressure in the opposite direction to that envisaged by the clinical effectiveness project team. For instance, a drug company may endeavour to promote H_2 antagonists rather than to encourage the use of eradication regimens.

Intensity of contribution required

Changing practice requires a lot of enthusiasm, hard work and long-term vision on the part of the project leaders.

PACE: The Lessons so far

A. Preparing the ground

Lesson A1. Base local guidelines on national reviews of evidence and guidelines.

Lesson A2. Acknowledge that evidence may be ambiguous and incomplete.

Lesson A3. Be clear about what needs to change.

Lesson A4. Link the work into local priorities.

Lesson A5. Consider the options available for securing change.

Lesson A6. Understand local issues and potential barriers to change.

Lesson A7. Take into account the needs and interests of GPs and primary health care teams.

Lesson A8. Establish data required to monitor progress.

B. Securing action

Lesson B1. Present the change in terms of benefits for staff and patients.

Lesson B2. Help people work together.

Lesson B3. Provide a local education and training programme.

Lesson B4. Give more than information to primary health care teams.

Lesson B5. A balanced approach across primary and secondary care is important.

Lesson B6. Decide how to engage pharmaceutical companies.

C. Managing the work

Lesson C1. Create a realistic timetable.

Lesson C2. Decide how to co-ordinate the work.

Lesson C3. Recognise that new skills may be required.

Lesson C4. Keep in touch with those affected by the work.

Lesson C5. Retain a balanced approach.

Lesson C6. Do not be too ambitious.

Lesson C7. Expect the unexpected and be able to respond.

Working with Primary Care

These notes supplement comments in Chapter 3. They are based on discussion with local projects about involving general practitioners and primary health care teams in their work and draw specifically on the projects in Bromley and North Derbyshire. The notes formed a special issue of the *PACE Bulletin* published in June 1997.

Work with primary care can usefully be considered under three broad headings:

- *Preparing and planning a work programme* that reflects the diversity of primary care

- Creating practical means of *engaging general practitioners and primary health care teams*

- Providing support to practices and *securing and sustaining change.*

Preparing and planning a work programme

Experience has shown that detailed preparation is essential to lay the ground for effective work with primary care. It is easy to be tempted to develop a plan of action that assumes that all practices are broadly the same. Such an approach is likely to fail. It is essential to recognise and build on the diversity of primary care. Practices will have their own interests and pressures – and it is unrealistic to expect them all to go forward at the same pace. They are each likely to have their own agenda and will raise different interests in debates about clinical effectiveness.

In developing a work programme it would be sensible to:

- Aim initially to tackle topics that are likely to be of importance and interest to primary care (North Derbyshire demonstrated that a high response to audit can be secured if the topic is initiated, led by and important to GPs)

- Think carefully about who has useful intelligence to help you engage GPs – people who know about their preferences – and explore ways to assemble that information

- Be incremental, create a programme to involve all practices gradually – not all at once; focus initially on those GPs who are likely to adopt new approaches

- Recognise that data collection in primary care may be difficult due to the lack of common information technology systems

- Identify resources to help practices with data collection (money or people)

It is also important to identify allies who will be able to reinforce the messages (but make sure they carry a consistent message!):

- Consultants willing to return inappropriate referrals based on guidelines

- GP tutors who will have knowledge of learning styles

- Community pharmacists who can reinforce prescribing advice

- Staff in health authorities (medical advisers, public health doctors and commissioning managers) who have contact with practices

- Staff involved in audit in primary and secondary care.

Engaging general practitioners and teams

The NHS is awash with paper so it is sensible to explore ways to build on existing channels for communications rather than create new arrangements – there are numerous newsletters, visits and professional meetings. Options for providing information to practices could also include seminars (set presentations followed by discussions), workshops (small group discussions), practice meetings (involving only local partners) and one-to-one meetings (academic detailing).

Care will be needed to establish which is the most suitable for each practice. Whatever course is adopted, PGEA recognition for the activity is helpful. Above all, find ways to make participation fun rather than business, try to finish meetings early and:

- Choose the time to approach practices with care and do not encroach on clinical contact time with patients (a lesson from Bromley – never ring a GP on a Monday!)

- Take the messages to GPs and practices on their home territory (North Derbyshire used a locality focus for all project activity)

- Invite practices to take part (North Derbyshire used this approach successfully for the initial audit and a quality of life survey)

- Consider carefully who should put their names to papers, letters and other documents – such as the MAAG chair, key local GPs, the director of public health or key local consultants (Bromley found it helpful to choose three: the MAAG chair, the director of public health and the consultant gastroenterologist)

- Avoid an adversarial approach (Bromley presented evidence, contrasted this with current practice and explored the scope for change (to practice) to demonstrate benefits; North Derbyshire used a district-wide audit).

Experience suggests that it is sensible to explore alternative routes into the primary health care team rather than relying solely on the GP. Other initial points of contact could be practice nurses and practice managers; the latter may be increasingly influential. If this course is adopted, bring in other members of the team as soon as possible. Whichever route is chosen, some of the projects' experiences about the content of the communications are:

- Keep messages simple – create simple standard notes, setting out what is involved, the benefits, what change may be required. Repeat messages regularly.

- Use language familiar to primary care – avoid management jargon and show understanding of the pressures and challenges in primary care. Acknowledge different terminology – some people like guidelines, others pathways or digests of evidence.

- Material, such as guidelines, needs to be visually appealing as well as practical and easy to use – and evidence-based! (North Derbyshire circulated 'PACE project practice packs'.)

- Presentation of information in a 'question and answer' format may be helpful.

- Explore ways to enhance the credibility of guidelines, remember GPs receive them from many quarters. How do they pick out which to follow?

- Guidelines need to have a 'valid until' date and should then be reviewed.

Securing and sustaining action

Reflecting the day-to-day pressures on primary health care teams it is unrealistic to expect the supply of information to change the nature of care and treatment provided to patients. The important point to get over is that the aim is to incorporate changes into routine clinical practice. In the medium term this may involve additional tasks but in the longer term effective practice should be professionally more rewarding as well as having a beneficial impact on patient outcomes. Experience has shown that some additional resources and support may be essential to initiate and help the process of change. For example, provide someone to work with the practice to identify existing patients whose care and treatment may require adjustment. Additional incentives could be:

- To ensure that any necessary service developments are in place – for example, adequate access to therapy or diagnostic services, before promoting the need for change to referral or treatment patterns

- To explore ways to cover reimbursement for locum costs – this works wonders to increase access to practices

- To present ways of securing a fast-track route to the consultant – for example, a new referral form or a dedicated telephone number

- To present the work in terms of its benefits to GPs as well as to patients. The Wirral schizophrenia project should take some pressure off GPs. The *H. pylori* and ulcer treatment projects should, in the longer term, reduce repeat prescriptions and eradicate peptic ulcer disease in a significant number of patients

- To create means of self-monitoring for practices – for example, identify simple measures that the health authority can provide to enable practices to achieve and maintain a sense of achievement (such as prescribing trends).

Effective Communications

These notes are based on discussion with some of the local projects about communication issues. The notes formed the main part of the PACE discussion paper *Effective Communications* (March 1997).

Using existing local networks

Effective communication needs to be maintained at a number of levels. Members of the core PACE project groups tend to maintain effective communication via informal face-to-face contact in-between formal meetings. However, ongoing communication between the core group, the steering group, the rest of the local health service and users needs more formal methods in order to ensure that the messages are disseminated regularly in a consistent and clear manner.

An example of a formal communications strategy comes from the Royal Berkshire and Battle Hospital's leg ulcer core project. The work on this project suggests that the stages involved in the implementation of the strategy are:

● Identification of all communication target groups including the (parent) steering group, relevant senior and 'ground' staff at acute and community trusts, primary health care teams, university departments, CHCs and user groups. It is particularly important to identify communication routes to target groups that do not have natural assemblies (like practice managers in primary care). The identification of all groups to target will help ensure that those harder-to-reach groups are not neglected. In addition, a database of parties that have shown an interest in the project could be established in order to ensure ongoing communication and harness enthusiasm

● Identification of existing communication routes and networks, such as newsletters, purchasing intentions, existing forums, educational events, user and community groups, health authority and trust board meetings. It is important to target communication routes that have high visibility

● Clarification of the agendas of the various professional and user groups. This is vital in order to appropriately tailor the messages given

● Identification of named people in the core PACE project group who would be responsible for the regular dissemination of information via identified communication routes. The core project group is multi-disciplinary. This provides a mechanism whereby group members communicate with members of their own professional or user group. The advantages of this are that they will already be aware of effective communication routes to that group. Also, they are likely to be known by members of the wider group, which facilitates informal dialogue and feedback. Table 1 above illustrates how the local PACE project core group assigns responsibility for

Target Audience	Routes
Community trust	
Neighbourhood managers	Nursing policy committee
District nurses	Tissue viability link nurses
GPs	Acute unit GP newsletter,
	MAAG open days
Acute trust	
CE and board	Board reports through director
CSU managers	Monthly nursing policy meeting
Ward sisters	Lead sisters' monthly meeting
Nursing staff	Practice development nurses,
Senior medical staff	tissue viability link nurses
PAMs	Postgraduate meetings
	Departmental meetings
Other local organisations	
University and college staff	College newsletter
Students on relevant courses	Course module leaders
Health authority	Commissioning meetings

Table 1 Responsibility for communications (examples only): a third column would show the initials of the appropriate member of the core group.

communications. To be effective the information needs to include all the target audiences, the current routes available and responsibility. It should be kept up to date at regular project group meetings

- Preparation of material, on a regular basis, appropriate for each communication route: detailed information packs on clinical effectiveness (particularly on the PACE project) for the steering group, update articles for the newsletter, relevant clinical vignettes for GP education forums and patient information leaflets

- Identification of mechanisms for measuring the effectiveness of the communication strategy – for example, measurement of response to invitations to study days advertised in local newsletters.

Creating special local events

The strategy described depends on existing routes of communication. However, it may also be necessary to hold additional events to stimulate debate on challenging issues.

These may include a large meeting held on an annual basis for all interested parties, including health workers, social services and user groups, to discuss progress. This could be followed by a special event incorporating workers in disciplines not previously involved in the project, but who could learn from lessons generalised from the work.

The PACE Project in Wirral, which involves the role of a family support worker (FSW), offers an example where special events have been helpful. This project relates to the employment of an FSW employed by a voluntary organisation (Making Space). It involves exploring issues about the links between the health authority, Making Space, the local NHS trusts, primary care and the local authority social services department. All the organisations have been open from the outset about their desired outcomes from the project and acknowledged that each agency had a different view. They recognised that the learning from the project work would help them reconcile these differences and the related tensions, and allow progress to be made.

A number of meetings were arranged with staff in the locality where the FSW operates, including GPs and other primary care staff, community psychiatric nurses, social services staff and ward staff relating to the area to ensure that people understand the role of the FSW and discuss how the FSW fits within the community mental health team. To supplement these meetings a programme of workshops is being arranged to explore a number of issues where learning from the project should contribute to the development of the role of the FSW.

The first workshop addressed issues including confidentiality and questions about the handling and sharing of information, team management, management of case record systems and the organisation and monitoring of assessment and review processes. The discussion provided the stimulus for a series of actions to help resolve the issues.

A second workshop is planned; the issues that need to be addressed include mechanisms for contracting with the voluntary sector, reconciling the differing policy objectives of the various organisations and agencies and the problems faced when a small organisation is working closely with larger teams and organisations.

Measuring Impact

These notes describe the principles that have been adopted to guide work on measurement within the PACE programme: they formed a part of the PACE discussion paper *Measuring Impact* (September 1996).

- Rely on *original research*. Given that PACE and other similar activities are concerned with implementing research-based, clinically effective programmes of care, there is no point in replicating primary research.

- Focus on the *process of implementation* rather than on researching health outcomes. Establishing health outcome is a complex and time-consuming process. Credible research material, including systematic reviews and meta analyses, is widely available and can be used to establish expected outcomes.

- Rely wherever possible on *routine data systems*. Creating customised data is often unnecessary given the wealth of information already available via routine data collection systems.

- Identify *suitable comparisons*. Finding true comparisons within the context of local project implementation is unlikely; nevertheless, it is still important to make some attempt to establish whether or not observed change has occurred as a direct result of the implementation.

- Establish a *baseline* against which to measure impact. Baseline information is important when attempting to establish the scale of change, and can also be used as a reference point from which to proceed. The baseline, which may be a rate or trend, might reflect norms at national, regional or local level.

- Build in a process to *monitor progress*. It is important to consider what is being measured, why it is being measured and how to measure it. These considerations will take into account the aims and objectives of the project, the availability and appropriateness of data – is a baseline available, are the data obtainable routinely, are they sensitive enough to detect progress?

Finally, keep it *as simple as possible*.

From Project to Mainstream

These notes are taken from the PACE discussion paper *From Project to Mainstream* (September 1996). The paper suggested steps that might be helpful in considering moving clinical effectiveness from project to mainstream.

Formulating a strategy

It may be helpful to see the task in three elements.

First, be alert to *precursors to change*, factors that can indicate a readiness for change, such as:

- Has the organisation an acknowledged set of values that supports the use of evidence in decision making, such as a collaborative, multi-professional style of working and a desire to do the right things (that is, deliver effective care)?

- Financial reality and other issues that might dominate the local management agenda

- Are those involved alert to the different funding and reporting channels (such as for professional education and audit) and different agendas?

- Are there benefits to those involved – how will the work help them provide better care?

- Recognition that research evidence may not provide clear-cut answers or address all aspects of care.

Second, identify and take a series of *steps to promote appropriate change* such as:

- Retaining a focus on a limited number of topics

- Promoting an incremental move from project to programme to mainstream

- Promoting shared learning between organisations, groups and functions

- Finding ways to provide help as well as information to clinicians

- Identifying product champions (in the key organisations, groups and functions)

- Being clear whether the aim is to change the way 'we' work or the way 'they' work – is the catalyst internal or external?

Third, develop a series of *markers of success* such as:

- Is the library or information service seen as a central resource for the organisation?

- Is there a clinical effectiveness programme addressing work on a range of topics and embracing the potential interests and contributions?

- Is there congruence between the work programmes of the different organisations groups and functions to improve the delivery of care?

- Are there productive relationships between clinical staff and managers?

- Are there training programmes that cross organisations, groups and functions?

- Is work on clinical effectiveness reflected in NHS contracts?

- Do corporate contracts and personal objectives cover clinical effectiveness, activity and results?

The PACE Network

Notes are circulated to participants in PACE Network discussion days. This is an example from one of the discussions, the Involving Patients discussion day on 24 April 1997. These notes are not intended to cover all the points that were raised on the day, but rather as a reminder of the main areas of discussion.

Participants were drawn from a wide range of organisations and while planning was in hand for a number of initiatives for involving patients, few had practical experience from completed work. Interest arose from desires to involve patients in a wide range of activities, including:

- Research studies, for example, a study of hospital re-admissions of elderly patients

- Treatment, for example, to ensure adherence to treatment plans

- Commissioning, for example, to guide the development of services for populations

- Audit projects, for example, to secure patients' contributions to set up and follow through projects.

While the focus was on issues related to health care, on a number of occasions we were reminded of the close links between health and social care. Close working with social services was therefore important. We structured the discussion under three broad headings: why involve patients?; how to involve patients; patient information.

Why involve patients?

We suggested that it was sensible, before projects were taken too far, to ensure that we ask whether we have a clear view about why we are involving patients and how we expect that involvement to influence the work.

A number of reasons were identified including:

- Policy imperatives – the Department expects it!

- To ensure that patients understand the likely impact of treatment and help to avoid the risk of litigation

- It could help to improve compliance. We heard about the examples of the development of care pathways that allow clinical staff to explain to patients the stages in their treatment and of contract treatment plans that record agreements between patients and chiropodists

- To help ensure that patients' views of outcomes are able to influence service development. This was important because much of the research about the effectiveness of health care reflected views on outcomes from a clinical or academic perspective

- Involvement in audit projects could ensure that standards are set to reflect patients' views of an effective service

- Patients rights, the work on the *Patient's Charter*, had given emphasis to rights of patients

- Patients can be experts in their condition. Patients offer a continuity of perspective beyond that of clinical staff.

How to involve patients

We spoke about the need for patient education to ensure that patients take more responsibility for their own health, and overcome some of the problems that arise because of their dependency on clinical staff. This required a balance with some initiatives best handled nationally to complement local initiatives.

Patients are likely to require advice and support to ensure that they are able to contribute effectively – this preparation may take time. Do not assume that you can just invite patients to group discussions and expect them to join in.

We identified a wide range of approaches that might be appropriate, including:

- Population surveys, although it was important to ensure that appropriate questions were used

- Focus groups and other patient groups

- Individual patients followed up as part of work on service quality

- Priority search techniques

- Better use of the intelligence that could be assembled from routine contacts between patients and clinical staff; at the moment this tends to be ignored if it constitutes a complaint

- Beware of only using a vocal minority. If one concern is about access to services, it may be more sensible to seek out patients who would not normally join in

- Contacts with CHC staff and members

- Working with self-help and other voluntary groups.

The important point was to ensure that the approach is appropriate to the task!

Patient information

- There are real problems at present because of the abundance of such material; it was difficult for NHS staff and patients to decide which leaflets and other items were the most reliable

- Start with quality material developed by others rather than starting from a blank sheet of paper

- The work on Promoting Patient Choice at the King's Fund and the Health Information Resource Centre in Winchester should in time provide useful support and advice. Many voluntary organisations have created material based on up-to-date evidence

- Ensure that patients have independent access to leaflets and other material; they should not be available only through clinical staff

- Leaflets should be backed up with one-to-one conversations between patients and clinicians to help ensure that patients understand the choices available or the treatment plan.